UNDERSTANDING
SEVERE ME

Essential Guide
For Family & Friends

By

C H Saunders
Former Severe ME Patient

Publishers' Note

This book has been written by Catherine Saunders who had Very Severe Myalgic Encephalopathy (ME) back in the late 90s/early 00s and is compiled from her personal experience of the illness and from talking to other Patients and their friends/relatives who have had first-hand experience of living with Severe ME.

The Author has **no** medical training, only her personal experience of having Severe ME. This book is intended only for guidance and information purposes; it is not intended to replace sound medical advice. The use of any information is entirely at the user's own risk.

Every ME/CFS Patient is unique and the Author strongly urges all Patients to always consult professional medical practitioners for a proper diagnosis, assessment and medical guidance before trying any of the treatments/ideas mentioned in this Book. As with all medications, Patients should always consult their GP, Specialist, and Pharmacist and tell them about other medications or herbal preparations they are taking; and they should always read the label and patient information leaflet.

Neither the Author nor the Publisher take responsibility for any possible consequences from any treatment, procedure, test, exercise, action or application of medication or preparation by any person reading or following the information in this book. The publication of this book does not constitute the practice of medicine, and this book does not attempt to replace your doctor.

First published in UK by Kindle Direct Publishing
©2017 C H Saunders
Text Copyright © C H Saunders 2017

A CIP catalogue record for this book is available from the British Library

ASIN (e-book): B077M8HNHD
ISBN (print edition): 9781973344452

Designed and typeset by: Word-2-Kindle with thanks to Nick Caya & Team

Foreword

By A J F Dutton, Carer

"ME/CFS is a cruel and physically disabling illness that wrecks lives, none more so than the extreme form of the illness: Severe ME. Few people understand or appreciate the true impact of this illness, and for the Families and Friends of Severe ME Patients, it can be a terrifying time.

Having been a Carer and Patient Advocate myself, I have first-hand experience of dealing with the frustration and fear that comes with this little-understood and much maligned disease. During that time, limited information was available and I spent a lot of time trying to explain to relatives and friends what was going on behind closed doors, time I simply did not have to spare.

This is the book I wish my Family and Friends could have read.

The Author, Catherine draws on her own inspirational Severe ME story to explain what is going on, what Patients and their Carers have to battle against every day, and how the understanding, support and compassion of Family and Friends can make a profound difference to a Patient's chances of improving.

It is an insightful, hopeful and easily accessible guide. Catherine addresses the many questions, worries and fears that Family and Friends have; sign-posts the way to expert sources of information and treatment areas, and most importantly, perhaps, suggests hundreds of ways that Family and Friends can help ease the burden for Patients and Carers, both practically and emotionally.

If you want to help and support a Severe ME Patient and their Carer(s), this is a book you need to read."

Author's Dedication

This book is dedicated firstly to my amazing husband who shared every moment of the nightmare with me; for his love, constancy and unerring faith which gave me the strength to fight on.

To my very special and precious mum, for always being there, and for your great friendship.

To Susan, for being the best mother-in-law a girl could wish for.

To all the friends and family who helped us through our hell on earth, too numerous to mention by name, but they know who they are. I truly would not have improved without your understanding, constancy and support.

To all the specialist medical professionals who helped me: Professor Findley, Jill Slorance and their wonderful team in Romford, Gill Walsh, Theresa Hawksworth, Tina Betts, Dr Downton, Dr Semple, Gayle Hillier, Ashley Meyer, Anne Dempsey, Nick Vine, Lin Du.

To all those who campaign fiercely on behalf of Severe ME Patients including: Action For ME, The ME Association, the 25% Group, Tymes Trust, ME Research UK, Stockport ME Group, Open Medicine Foundation, and Jennifer Brea for making the amazing film, Unrest, that reveals the true horror of Severe ME. And lastly, but by no means least, to Kay Gilderdale and in memory of her daughter, Lynn, and all the Severe ME Patients we have tragically lost. I truly hope they have all found peace at last.

Contents

Introduction

"The physical symptoms can be as disabling as multiple sclerosis, systemic lupus erythematosus, rheumatoid arthritis and other chronic conditions..."

National Institute for Health and Clinical Excellence
Clinical Guideline 53, Page 3 Quick Reference Guide
Chronic fatigue syndrome/myalgic encephalomyelitis (or encephalopathy)
Diagnosis and management of CFS/ME in adults and children

Myalgic Encephalomyelitis **(ME),** also known as Chronic Fatigue Syndrome **(CFS)** or **ME/CFS**, is a devastating, physically disabling, multi-system disease that causes dysfunction of the neurological, immune, endocrine and energy metabolism systems. It often follows an infection and leaves 75% of those affected unable to work and 25% severely affected. An estimated 15-30 million people worldwide have ME.

Whatever the name, it is an illness that devastates lives and none more so than the lives of those severely affected.

Severe ME is not as rare as you might think.

As you can see from the figures below, the number of people in the UK with Severe ME is not that far behind the number of people with Multiple Sclerosis (MS) or HIV in the U.K.

However, the medical support/treatments available are a million miles behind those offered to MS and HIV Patients.

<u>Approx. Number of people in UK having:</u>

ME (all levels)   250,000   (Source www.afme.org.uk 2017)
Of which approx 25%:
Severe ME   62,500   (Source www.afme.org.uk 2017

| Multiple Sclerosis | 107,740 | (Source www.mssociety.org.uk 2016) |
| HIV | 101,200 | (Source www.avert.org 2015) |

The National Institute for Health and Care Excellence (NICE) acknowledges that the physical symptoms of ME can be as disabling as multiple sclerosis, systemic lupus erythematosus, rheumatoid arthritis, congestive heart failure and other chronic conditions. Other research shows that people with ME score lower overall on health-related quality of life tests than most other chronic conditions (Hvidberg et al, 2015).

Due to the sterling work of ME bodies such as AFME, The 25% Group, ME Research UK, Tymes Trust and The ME Association, awareness of Severe ME **is** building and the situation is not quite as bleak as it once was – specialist NHS medical teams are being developed, and help is getting to some Patients; **but** I am still constantly shocked and dismayed by how few people in the UK really understand and appreciate the true impact of this illness.

Before I became ill, I used to think ME was just about being tired. How blissfully ignorant I was. Severe ME may not be a terminal illness, but it takes people's lives; I know, because it took mine for several years. For the best part of 2 years I was a breathing corpse. For 15 months I did not see daylight, so severe was my light sensitivity. All I could do was lay in a blacked-out room in constant pain, unable to talk or walk. I had to be fed, watered, washed, dressed and nursed by my husband and family, just like a baby.

And one of my promises to myself whilst I was so severely affected, was to do all I could, when I could, no matter how long it took me, to help family/friends of Severe ME Patients understand just what it is that their loved one is going through; what Patients and their Carers have to battle against every day, and how their understanding, compassion and support can make such a dramatic difference to the their chances of improving.

Indeed, *understanding* is perhaps one of the greatest 'gifts' people can give to Severe ME Patients and if this Book prevents just one Patient/Carer from wasting scarce energies convincing others of the physically disabling nature of this illness, then I will have achieved my goal. Over the coming pages I will try to explain the harsh reality of Severe ME, address the many questions, worries and fears about what is happening to your friend/relative and suggest ways in which you may ease their burden.

Severely affected ME Patients can improve, but only if they are given the right advice, the right treatments, the right support, at the right time – always remember that, no matter how bad things get for your loved one, they can escape the hell of Severe ME, in time, and regain some quality of life; just try to be there for them and their Carers – listen to them, learn along with them, support them – you really can make a difference.

My heart goes out to everyone affected by Severe ME, wherever you live in the world. Whether you are a patient, carer, relative or friend, I truly hope you find this Guide helpful

Heaps of love and strength,

Catherine

Website: www.understandingsevereme.blogspot.co.uk
Email: understandingsevereme@hotmail.co.uk

Chapter 1: The Different Levels of ME

"Every illness affects people differently, affecting some severely, some more mildly...you only have to think of think of Cancer, Heart Disease, Multiple Sclerosis. Why is it then so difficult for people to understand that this range and degree of illness also occurs in ME?

People diagnosed with Cancer, Heart Disease, MS receive so much compassion and understanding from people...and rightly so...but why do people affected by Severe ME not receive that same level of support when they too are suffering?"

Susan Firth Dutton
Carer of Severe ME Patient

The National Institute for Health and Clinical Excellence (NICE) categorises the different levels of ME as follows *(source NICE Clinical Guideline 53, August 2007):*

'Severity

*   *People with **Mild CFS/ME** are mobile, can take care of themselves and do light domestic tasks with difficulty. Most are still working or in education but to do this they have probably stopped all leisure and social pursuits, and often take days off.*

*   *People with **Moderate CFS/ME** have reduced mobility and are restricted in all activities of daily living, although they may have peaks and troughs in their level of symptoms and ability to do activities. They have usually stopped work or education and need rest periods. Their sleep at night is generally poor quality and disturbed.*

*   *People with **Severe CFS/ME** are unable to do any activity for themselves, or can carry out minimal daily tasks only (such as face washing, cleaning teeth). They have Severe cognitive*

difficulties and depend on a wheelchair for mobility. They are often unable to leave the house, or have a Severe and prolonged after-effect if they do so. They may also spend most of their time in bed, and are often extremely sensitive to light and noise.'

Having been very severely affected I agree with those who believe that the 'Severe' category needs to be broken down further, into *'Severe ME'* and *'Very Severe ME'*. It is vital that people understand that a Very Severely Affected Patient is TOTALLY DEPENDENT upon their carer(s).

So below is an excerpt from Diane L Cox's book *Occupational Therapy and Chronic Fatigue Syndrome*, which explains the levels of ability in ME Patients very clearly:

'Levels of Ability

Patients with CFS can present with a wide range of symptoms and levels of ability. For ease of identifying the type of management approach required, the patients referred to the hospital are divided into four levels of ability. The levels were devised so that each patient is categorized dependent upon level of fatigue, daily activity level and general mobility (Cox, 1998; Cox and Findley, 1998):

- Mild (Grade 1)
- Moderate (Grade 2)
- Severe (Grade 3)
- Very Severe (Grade 4)

*The patients in the **mild** category will be mobile and self-caring and able to manage light domestic and work tasks with extreme difficulty. The majority will still be working. However, in order to remain in work, they will have stopped all leisure and social pursuits, often taking days off. Most will use the weekend to rest in order to cope with the week.*

*The patients in the **moderate** category will have reduced mobility and be extremely restricted in all activities of daily living, often having* *peaks and troughs of ability, dependent on the degree of symptoms. The patients in this group have usually stopped work and require many rest periods, often sleeping in the afternoon for one to two hours. Sleep quality at night is generally poor and disturbed. This level appears to be the group most cited in the description of studies and CFS services (Cox and Findley, 1994; Wilson et al., 1994b; Sharpe et al., 1996; Vercoulen et al., 1996; Deale et al., 1997; Fulcher and White, 1997).*

The patients in the **severe** *category will be able to carry out minimal daily tasks only, such as face washing and cleaning teeth, have severe cognitive difficulties and be wheelchair dependent for mobility. These patients are often unable to leave the house except on rare occasions with a severe prolonged after-effect from effort.*

The patients in the **very severe** *category will be unable to mobilise or carry out any daily task for themselves and are bed-bound for the majority of the time. These patients are often unable to tolerate any noise, and are generally extremely sensitive to light.'*

Occupational Therapy and Chronic Fatigue Syndrome,
(Page 80-81) by Diane L Cox

As you can see, the difference between the levels is huge, just as in any illness.

Perhaps the reason that Severe ME and Very Severe ME are so poorly understood is that mainstream media mostly concentrates on Patients with Mild/Moderate ME, the 'walking wounded', who are able to be interviewed, are seen by people up and about on their good days, and are able to attend out Patient clinics.

Whereas those who are Severely* affected do indeed become 'invisible'; left bed-bound, little more than breathing corpses, they cannot speak for themselves to explain to the World what this illness is really like; they cannot access appropriate specialist medical care, because both in-Patient and domiciliary care is still scarce; and they cannot be included in the research studies because, they are too physically disabled to take part.

* As you read this pack, please bear in mind that for conciseness sake, whenever I use the term 'Severe ME', I am indeed including within that term Very Severe ME Patients too.

Chapter 2: Severe ME Causes and Triggers

Unfortunately, there is still, at the time of writing, no simple, definitive answer as to what causes Severe/Very Severe ME and until the massive under-researching of this wholly debilitating illness is corrected, sadly, that will remain the case.

However, we Patients and Carers have to find ways to explain to ourselves and our family and friends what is going on; and during my illness and ongoing recovery journey, I have trawled the internet, read myriad books and hundreds of articles, trying to understand this bewildering illness.

I am no medical expert, but I am an expert in my illness, and how I try to explain Severe ME to my family and friends; I try to focus their minds upon what I believe to be the biggest pieces in the causal jigsaw so here is how I explain what is happening to Severe ME Patients:

1.   Genetic predisposition to contracting Severe ME

2.   A triggering event or infection eg viral damage to body/brain at a time when the person is under immense stress

3.   Immune System 'crash'/ dysfunction

4.   Dysfunction of Central and Autonomic Nervous Systems

5.   Hypothalamus/Pituitary/Adrenal axis dysfunction

6.   Mitochondrial dysfunction
      (Mitochondria are the tiny structures that generate energy within cells)

7. Deficit of oxygen in the brain stem

8. Major 'power cut' to body/brain leading effectively to 'paralysis from within'

Chapter 3: What is going on?

"...This virus competes with the body for energy, entering mitochondria (the energy-producing power stations inside cells) and destroying them. Thus, the body has a major power failure since mitochondria produce maximum energy in the body. When there is a power failure, every organ and system become sluggish and the body becomes 'paralysed' from within. This is the Severest form of CFS. The presence of the virus in the tonsils and lymphatic glands causes frequent feverish sensations, swelling of glands and so on.

Such Patients are barely able to move, as muscles, which have an abundance of mitochondria, become inert and lifeless. They ache because the mitochondria are unable to burn glucose properly and so lactic acid accumulates in them..."

Dr Mosaraf Ali
The Integrated Health Bible

So, what do we know? Around 66%* of ME cases are **triggered by a viral infection** such as flu, glandular fever, Epstein Barr, meningitis, hepatitis; indeed, my own illness was triggered by a recurrent bout of tonsillitis, treated again by antibiotics at a time when I was under a lot of **stress** at work. (*AFME statistic)

Other less common triggers include bacterial infection; exposure to toxins in the environment; an immunization given to a person whilst unwell; physical trauma or injury, such as an accident or operation; increased stress combined with one of the factors above.

Studies have shown that ME affects many body systems, in particular the **Immune System** and the **Central Nervous System (CNS).** Indeed, The World Health Organisation classifies ME/CFS as a disease of the CNS, the same category in which it places Multiple Sclerosis and Parkinson's Disease.

It seems that after the initial viral attack on the body, ME Patients' immune systems go into some kind of 'overdrive', excessive levels of **cytokines** (killer cells) are produced, the genes in Patients' white blood cells – a key part of the immune system – are switched on and off in an abnormal fashion and the **Hypothalamic-Pituitary-Adrenal axis (HPA)**, part of your Central Nervous System, is affected. The Hypothalamus is the major gland of the body, governing practically every system, organ and function – the effects of its dysfunction upon the body/brain of a Patient are Severe.

Staying with how the Central Nervous System is affected, it appears that in ME Patients, the **Sympathetic Nervous System is more easily activated and can be predominant nearly all the time** *(in Professor Findley's words - abnormal stress response system).*

Outlined below is information that was kindly explained to me during my time with the CFS/ME Unit at Old Church Hospital, Romford, Essex, back in 2002, which helped me really understand what was going on in my body and brain:

AUTONOMIC NERVOUS SYSTEM*

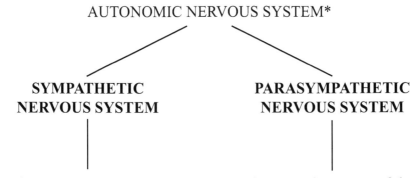

SYMPATHETIC NERVOUS SYSTEM

PARASYMPATHETIC NERVOUS SYSTEM

Produces a stress reaction. An essential Survival mechanism where large amounts of energy can be accessed for short term use. In the wild it has enabled us to give our best in either fighting or running away. A 'fight or flight' response.

Produces a calm or peaceful effect. Essential for convalescence, healing and reorganising. Energy is directed and resourced in a long-term way to enable performance of self-Nurturing activities.

With a Severe ME Patient basically 'stuck' in the stressful 'fight or flight' state almost permanently, their primary body systems are greatly affected:

STRESSED Patient	BODY SYSTEM	CALM PATIENT
Rapid breathing, from upper part of chest	BREATHING	Breathing is slow and from lower part of chest, using Diaphragm
Blood directed to brain, which is working overtime in a problem Manner	CIRCULATION OF BLOOD	Blood is directed to skin and and digestive system – skin is warm and digestion improved
Muscles tense and ready for action	MUSLES & JOINTS	Muscles relaxed, pressure taken off joints
Senses are on high alert eg, hearing straining to pick up slightest sound that will aid fight or flight	SPECIAL SENSES	Senses reduced, eg sounds seem quieter, more distant
Digestion switched off as body prepares for Fight or flight.	DIGESTION	Digestion switched on, working efficiently
The brain is working over-time in a problem solving manner, to make sure that around you and to help you cope with any problems that may occur	BRAIN	Thoughts become unfocused and creative with a day dream quality you are aware of everything

SYMPATHETIC ------------ ● ------------ **PARASYMPATHETIC**
(STRESS)   (CALM)

The two systems behave like a see-saw, one side in predominance whilst the other is quiet. The aim, therefore, for ME Patients, is to identify ways of gaining control of the see-saw and access the Parasympathetic Nervous System.

Dr Sarah Myhill, a leading ME specialist, (www.drymhill.co.uk) who has successfully treated thousands of ME Patients over the last 25 years, has long suspected that in ME there is a generalised **mitochondrial cell failure** *(ref Interaction Issue 56 www.afme.org. uk)*; and Dr Jonathan Kerr of Imperial College, London, undertook research into the **genes** of people with ME to try and understand the root causes of our illness. 15 genes were identified, which are different in ME Patients, involving the immune system, neurological function and mitochondrial function:

'.... He (Jonathan Kerr) said the results support a theory that the condition is often triggered by viruses such as Epstein-Barr, Q fever, enteroviruses and parvovirus B19, which causes lasting changes in gene expression that lead to chronic fatigue.

"CFS/ME often begins with a flu-like illness which never goes away", *Dr Kerr said.*

Many of the genes identified as different affect the functioning of the ***mitochondria*** *– the tiny structures that generate energy within cells.*

"The involvement of such genes does seem to fit with the fact that these (ME) Patients lack energy and suffer from fatigue" '

The Times
Thursday July 21

More recently, ground breaking research is being undertaken by The Open Medicine Foundation (OMF) in America whose mission is to fund and initiate collaborative research designed to find biomarkers and effective treatments for ME/CFS. OMF now has world renowned scientist, Ron Davies, on board, helping the team to find a diagnostic biomarker and effective treatments; and Prof Ron Davis is more driven than most as his own poor son, Whitney, is very severely affected. For Ron Davis, this is personal: it is a race to see if he can make significant progress in time to save his son, his heartbreak and frustration shared and understood by every parent who too is looking after a Severe ME patient and watching them suffer. (www.omf.ngo)

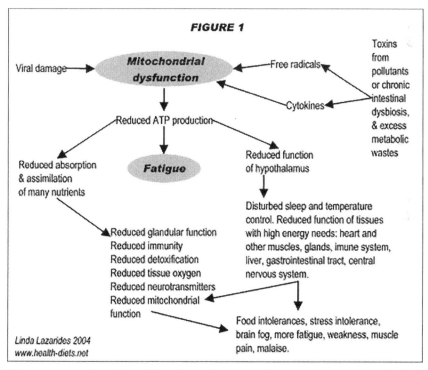

ATP: adenosine triphosphate, the name given to raw energy made by the mitochondria

Dysbiosis: overgrowth of harmful bacteria or fungi (eg candida) in the small intestine.

Mitochondria: the part of the cell which makes ATP (energy)

Linda Lazarides
Interaction
www.afme.org.uk

So, at long last, the mitochondria are finally getting some serious attention in ME/CFS research and with OMF specifically conducting large scale research into the Severe ME Patients Group via the OMF *ME/CFS Severely Ill Big Data Study*, finally the situation looks more promising for this group of patients long ignored and abandoned by the medical profession. But whilst we wait for news, we still need to try and explain what the hell is going on to our nearest and dearest.

Linda Lazarides, a top nutritional health expert, wrote an enlightening article in which she used a great diagram to illustrate what she believes is happening in ME Patients, which I have often used to show family and friends what is happening to Severe ME Patients.

But why are some Patients only mildly affected whilst others become so very severely affected?

For some individuals it is sadly the harsh hand that fate has dealt them – in much the same way that some people get terminal Cancer whilst other Cancer Patients make full recoveries, or some people get Type I Diabetes whilst others get Type II Diabetes, or some people have fatal Heart Attacks whilst others recover fully from a Mild Heart Attack.

Progress **is** being made in the NHS' specialist ME services, but I believe that, **historically**, the majority of Severe ME Patients became so Severely affected because they had been let down by the medical world. Either they had not been diagnosed quickly enough and/or not given the appropriate advice and treatment so necessary to give them any chance of recovery. Most commonly, uninformed medical professionals pushed ME Patients to their limits when they should have urged them to rest, throw their hands up in horror when the Patient takes a turn for the worse and then abandon them as they have no idea how to help them.

Take my case for example. Aged 32 – happily married, successful career, active, sporty – saw the onset of Moderate ME after a recurrent bout of tonsillitis treated by antibiotics. Luckily my original GP correctly and swiftly diagnosed ME; unluckily she gave me neither individual guidance nor individual treatment, but sent me to a group out-patient ME management programme run by a Clinical Psychologist at my local NHS Hospital. For 2 hours per week, for 9 weeks, 8 Mild/Moderate ME Patients, (the 'walking wounded'), each with a totally unique set of symptoms, received the same general advice.

At the end of the course, during my **only** one to one session, the Psychologist totally dismissed a fellow Patient's advice to me to be extremely cautious, and then went on to reassure and encourage me to be positive and attempt a return to work on a part time basis. I heeded her 'go for it' advice – she was the (supposed) ME expert after all; but she pushed my body and my brain too far, too fast, resulting in my collapsing 1 week later; and once my body had been put under so much physical stress I was in an unstoppable downward spiral, deteriorating rapidly into very Severe ME

Moral of the story for medical professionals: **advise ME patients to be cautious tortoises not hasty hares.**

Chapter 4: How bad can Severe ME get?

"Before meeting this remarkable mother and daughter I had seen African children suffering from starvation, met people dying of Aids, patients paralysed from the neck down, others in the last stages of terminal cancer. But I had never seen a living person as desperately ill as Lynn Gilderdale.

Hypersensitive to light and noise, she lay on a sheepskin to prevent bedsores, with her head resting on a towel. There was a tube down her nose delivering liquid food and a Hickman line pumping drugs straight into her chest. Her legs were paralysed and without feeling, she was unable to sit up without passing out and her neck was too weak to support her head.

She had lost more than half the bone density in her spine and had gone through the menopause at the age of 20. She was in constant pain. She was on drugs to prevent sickness and spasms, was unable to swallow and had not spoken since August 1992, three months after she had been diagnosed with ME at the age of 14.

In my 35 years as a journalist, the story of Lynn and Kay Gilderdale was one of the most affecting cases I had come across. I felt shocked, chastened and humbled as I talked to them and the memory of Lynn's haunting brown eyes, set in an exquisitely beautiful face, has stayed with me ever since"

Gill Swain, Daily Mail, Tuesday, December 9
Written after Lynn's death from a morphine overdose

62,500 people are estimated to fall into the 'Severe ME' category. This category in itself covers both Severely Affected Patients and Very Severely Affected Patients – and indeed the term 'bed-bound' can itself have a range of meanings, from the Patient who can still sit up in bed to feed themselves, right through to those Patients who have to be spoon fed, put on a drip, or tube fed.

Severely affected Patients do tend to become invisible. Only their Carer(s) see the harsh reality of this disabling illness first hand, but if you really want to help your relative/friend and support their Carer(s), **you** need to gain a detailed insight into the symptoms that they have to endure day in day out, and the level of disability that they face 24/7.

As you read the tables in the next chapter, keep reminding yourself that these symptoms last not for a few days, a few weeks or a few months – but maybe for a couple of years. All the activities that normal people just take for granted are ripped from Patients' lives. For example, I was unable to walk to our toilet for 2 years, having to rely on bedpans/commodes/chemical loo in the bedroom; I was unable to enjoy a shower for 3 years, having to rely on weekly bed-baths from my husband; I was unable to feed myself for 1 year, having to be spoon fed; I was unable to read, write, watch TV, or listen to the radio for 2 ½ years, having to just lay in bed, visualising myself well, willing my body to start to improve.

So, the next time you hear someone say that ME is just about being a bit tired, please feel free to correct them.

Common Severe ME Symptoms:

• Chronic pain – may be muscular, joint, neuropathic, headache (often migrainous)

• Severe, persistent and disabling fatigue of a type entirely distinct from everyday tiredness. This fatigue feels like being **paralysed from within**

• Delayed fatigue, often experienced up to 72 hours after a simple exertion, which is not made better by rest. Sufferers may take days/weeks/months to recover from a delayed fatigue episode.

• Neurological impairments including paralysis, seizures, muscles spasms, involuntary muscle movement and blackouts.

- Muscle weakness.

- Cognitive impairments such as brain fog – difficulty in concentration, problems with memory and attention span, difficulties with word-finding, planning/organising thoughts and information processing.

- Difficulty with sleep patterns, such as insomnia, hypersomnia, un-refreshing sleep and disturbed sleep-wake cycle.

- Increased sensitivity to sensory stimuli such as light or sound.

- Postural hypotension or rotational dizziness.

- Feeling too hot or cold – a problem with temperature control.

- Irritable Bowel like symptoms.

- Recurrent sore throat and/or enlarged lymph glands

Chapter 5: How does Severe ME affect Patients' daily lives?

"......People with CFS. are as sick and as functionally impaired as someone with AIDS, with breast cancer, with chronic obstructive pulmonary disease," said Dr William Reeves, the lead expert on the illness at the C.D.C. (Center for Disease Control and Prevention,"

Excerpt from New York Times, July 17
Frontline Report 'Chronic Fatigue No Longer Seen as 'Yuppie Flu'
By David Tuller

Outlined in the tables that follow is a breakdown of how each aspect of a Patient's life can be affected by Severe ME (referred to as CFS. above), both physically and cognitively.

Study these tables, really think about what you are reading, and really try and imagine what it must be like to have to live this nightmare:

PHYSICAL EFFECTS	SEVERE ME PATIENTS	VERY SEVERE ME PATIENTS
Toileting:	Commodes/Bedpans the norm. May be able to use standard toilet occasionally with Carers' help and/or using a seat to go over toilet to raise it.	Catheterised or lifted on/off bedpans by Carer. Plastic/waterproof sheets on bed and/or incontinence pads through night Independent toileting impossible.
Body Washing	Bath/shower may be possible with help of Carer, probably only once or twice a month; bath seats/hoists necessary. Patient may be able to use baby wipes independently or a bowl of water by bed/commode eg once a week.	Showers/Baths impossible. Face/hands/private parts washed eg weekly by Carers, moving bed-bound Patients limbs for them as they lay immobile. A full/half body wash may only be possible by Carers eg monthly, moving Patients limbs for them as they lay immobile. Showers impossible.

PHYSICAL EFFECTS	SEVERE ME PATIENTS	VERY SEVERE ME PATIENTS
Hair Washing	Only possible with help of Carer, probably only once or twice a month using bath seat/hoist over bath. Dry shampoo useful if Patient not allergic/sensitive to ingredients. Unable to neither brush/comb hair nor use hairdryer.	Every couple of months, Carers may be able to lift/roll Patient so head hangs over end of bed. Carer places plastic sheets underneath head/shoulders and washes hair using bottles of warm water, allowing water to run off into bucket on floor. This only possible if pain in neck, head and shoulders manageable. Unable to use neither hairbrush/comb nor hairdryer.
Brushing Teeth	May be possible independently with use of electric toothbrush, usually using a bowl/towel by bed	Carried out by Carers as Patient lays with mouth open & protective sheet/towel over Patient. Some Patients will not be able to tolerate the noise of an electric toothbrush Due to their noise sensitivity (see below)

PHYSICAL EFFECTS	SEVERE ME PATIENTS	VERY SEVERE ME PATIENTS
Eating & Drinking	*May be able to feed self if lying down or propped up on pillows.*	*Spoon fed by Carers as Patient lays with mouth open.*
	Food will need to be cut up/ casseroled/mashed/liquidised for Patient and usually; they will only be able to use a spoon to self-feed. Often alternating hands to hold the spoon, 1 mouthful with right, next with left etc, so helping the arms muscles to cope.	*Digestive system Severely affected so food usually has to be casseroled/mashed/ pureed/liquidised.*
		Some Patients who are unable to chew/swallow, or just too weak or whose digestion is very Severely affected; have to be Tube-fed.
	Feeding requires a lot of precious energy from the Patient, so little and often is the way, pacing eating throughout the day.	*Carers help Patient sip drinks with aid of straw.*
	May be able to pick up a glass/ bottle and drink independently	*Patient may be able to drink independently if eg water bottle left next to head on pillow along with straw; Patient unscrews cap, leans head to one side as unable to lift bottle, and drinks through straw.*

PHYSICAL EFFECTS	SEVERE ME PATIENTS	VERY SEVERE ME PATIENTS
Digestion	Digestive system greatly affected. Allergies, intolerances, constipation, nausea, bloating and diarrhoea very common. Need to eat little and often to help stabilise blood sugar levels. Hypoglycaemic attacks are common and terrifying as Patient can just pass out at any time.	Digestion may be so Severely affected that Tube Feeding is the only way to get food and nutrients into the Patient. If able to tolerate easy to swallow meals by being spoon fed, meals need to be little and often to help control hypoglycaemic attacks.
Cooking	Very limited ability, eg cut up an apple, butter a rice cake or maybe peel some vegetables for Carer to cook – arms just so easily fatigued. Also, so exhausting for most Patients to sit more than a few minutes at a time.	Totally unable
Dressing	Very limited ability eg put on a sock.	Totally unable

PHYSICAL EFFECTS	SEVERE ME PATIENTS	VERY SEVERE ME PATIENTS
	Most Patients unable to raise arms over head to put on clothes, so limbs usually lifted/lowered by Carer. *Necessity dictates choice of clothes eg when I could walk 12 paces once daily to loo, I was too weak to bend to pull PJ bottoms down, so had to have the bum cut out of them – undignified yes, but not as bad as a bedpan!*	*Will have to be dressed/undressed by Carer, limbs lifted/lowered by Carer due to Patient's physical disability*
Sitting	*May be able to be propped up in bed into a semi-sitting position, using pillows for support.* *May be able to sit in a chair, for short periods of time, eg starting at 1-2 minutes, best if chair is high*	*Totally unable independently. Unable to sit in chair. Unable to even prop self up on pillows.* *May be able to be propped up in bed by Carer for a few minutes each day, using pillows to support limbs, eg 3-4 pillows behind head and shoulders,*

PHYSICAL EFFECTS	SEVERE ME PATIENTS	VERY SEVERE ME PATIENTS
	backed with arms to give body support. Pillows used to make limbs comfortable and minimise pain. May need Carers help to get in/out of chair.	2 pillows under knees and 1 pillow over chest to support arms Pressure sores can develop if Patient lays in same position for long time. Carer needs to change Patients position slightly, say 3 hourly; District Nurse will be able to organise a special pressure relieving mattress or a motorised bed which can be raised/ lowered to change Patients position more easily.
Standing	Severely limited ability. Limbs/body/muscles wholly unable to produce energy required. Dizziness on standing very common.	Totally unable.

PHYSICAL EFFECTS	SEVERE ME PATIENTS	VERY SEVERE ME PATIENTS
	Joint pain (knee, ankle, hips) Severe when Patient tries to stand.	
	May be able to stand for short period IF supported by Carer, but pain and dizziness often prevent even that.	
	When Severely affected, I could manage to stand for 10 seconds once a day, then gradually increased standing time by 5 seconds when able.	
Walking in house	*Severely limited ability.*	*Totally unable.*
	Limbs/body/muscles wholly unable to produce energy required.	
	If Patient attempts to walk eg 20 paces to commode, support from Carer and/or from walking sticks,	

PHYSICAL EFFECTS	SEVERE ME PATIENTS	VERY SEVERE ME PATIENTS
	crutches, Zimmer frames, or from leaning on furniture/walls, necessary; *When Severely affected, I could walk 4 paces to a commode 4 times daily by holding onto wall for balance, and then began to increase number of trips when able.*	
Walking outside house	*Totally unable.*	*Totally unable.*
Stairs	*Totally unable.* *May be able to use a stairlift with Carer's help or be carried upstairs/downstairs by Carer if pain allows.*	*Totally unable.*

PHYSICAL EFFECTS	SEVERE ME PATIENTS	VERY SEVERE ME PATIENTS
Wheelchair in house	*If supported by pillows in wheelchair, Patient may be able to sit in wheelchair for very short periods, and be pushed around house by Carer.*	*Totally unable.*
Excursions in wheelchair	*Severely limited ability.* *Excursions demand huge amounts of energy, both physical and cognitive, so are attempted only with extreme caution, and usually only out of necessity.* *If Patient strong enough and the activity does not trigger setback, Carer pushing Patient in wheelchair around garden may be possible.*	*Totally unable.*

PHYSICAL EFFECTS	SEVERE ME PATIENTS	VERY SEVERE ME PATIENTS
Excursions in car	Attempted only out of extreme necessity, eg admission to specialist ME unit in hospital, but only if able to lay down in car or travel by ambulance. Car vibrations can really exacerbate the muscle/joint pain of Patient. If journey attempted, Patient will have to wear black out eye mask and ear plugs to prevent sensory overload/migraine from noise/light, and be cushioned by several pillows/mattress to reduce muscle/joint pain.	Totally Unable.
Talking	Patient may be able to whisper or mouth words for carer to lip read.	Patients often unable to speak and some may be paralysed.

PHYSICAL EFFECTS	SEVERE ME PATIENTS	VERY SEVERE ME PATIENTS
	Unable to shout out to a Carer, Patient will need other 'summoning' aids eg	*Their only communication may be 1 blink of the eyes for yes, 2 blinks of the eyes for no.*
	- Baby monitor listening device by bed, linked to a monitor carried around in house by Carer: *- a little bell to ring for help* *- a whistle around neck to blow for help*	*If Patient able to tolerate light, and can point, Carers can make Patient a Board with important words on eg hungry, thirsty, cold, hot, wee, poo, yes, no, etc, so that the Patient can point as needs;* *A Board with letters of the alphabet also useful for Patient to point at to communicate.*
	For Patients strong enough to use one, a mobile phone can be a great aid, with landline number; Carer's mobile/work number programmed in for speed dial; this is a great help for those Patients who are on their own for long periods of time.	*If Patient light sensitive and has to lay in darkened room, Patient uses fingers/hands to communicate eg 1 hand squeeze for yes, 2 hand squeezes for no, and hold 1 finger for bedpan, 2 fingers for hungry, 3 fingers for thirsty, 4 fingers for medication*

Personal Care

Just a quick word on the area of Personal Care. It is hard for normal healthy people to contemplate not being able to have a shower, bath or wash on a daily basis or being unable to use the toilet independently. For Severe ME Patients, however, Body Washing, Hair Washing and Toileting use such huge amounts of scarce and precious energy that to attempt them regularly simply leads to further physical deterioration and the slowing of their body's recovery process. At my most Severe, when my body simply could not produce the energy it needed to function, I went for 2 years unable to walk the 12 paces to the toilet, not even once a day, having to use a pee pot/commode/bedpan instead; and over 3 years without a shower, relying on baby wipes and a fortnightly bed-bath by my Carers – I find it hard now to imagine being so physically disabled, but I do vividly remember that when we attempted a daily bed-bath, and a weekly hair wash, the pain and the exhaustion of being moved/turned over/touched was crippling, leaving me feeling literally paralysed for days, sometimes unable to move any part of my body except my eyes. Utterly terrifying.

By conserving my precious energies, diverting those energies involved in personal care to the job of helping my body/brain concentrate on starting to self-correct, I know that I facilitated my recovery – I discovered that, if necessary, it is fine to go for at least a month or more without having my entire body/ hair washed – it sounds horrible, but being squeaky clean just was not worth it, my recovery was. Bear this in mind before you start criticising Carers or thinking that the Patient is just not trying hard enough.

COGNITIVE EFFECTS:	SEVERE ME PATIENTS	VERY SEVERE ME PATIENTS
Insomnia	*Same as very Severe ME Patient, but slightly less so.*	*Sleep cycle very Severely affected; at one extreme Patient may sleep egg 18-20 hours a day or at the other end of the spectrum and more commonly, Patient sleeps very little eg only 3-4 hours a night, and even that short amount usually restless and un-refreshing.*

COGNITIVE EFFECTS:	SEVERE ME PATIENTS	VERY SEVERE ME PATIENTS
		Many relatives/friends assumed that being bed-bound meant that I slept most of the time. How I wish!
		One of the most frustrating parts of very Severe ME is that the Patient's brain is in some kind of 'hyper' mode, whirring, buzzing, constantly, and most usually, at night when the Patient is desperate to sleep but unable to switch off the brain. Another symptom resulting primarily from dysfunction of Patient's autonomic nervous system.
		Patient stuck in vicious cycle of total exhaustion, no sleep, total exhaustion, no sleep, total exhaustion, no sleep....
Light Sensitivity	*Increased sensitivity to Light common.*	*Very increased sensitivity to light.*
		Can last for months and in some cases, years.

COGNITIVE EFFECTS:	SEVERE ME PATIENTS	VERY SEVERE ME PATIENTS
	Can last for months and in some cases, years.	*Patient often has to wear eye mask, have blackout curtains at windows, and no artificial light in room.*
	Exposure to light results in physically debilitating migraines/ nausea.	*Exposure to any light results in physically disabling and terrifyingly painful migraines and/ or nausea, dizziness, which can last for days and sometimes weeks.*
	Standard coping techniques include eye masks, blackout curtains, no normal lighting in room and Carers regularly having to navigate room in dark, or at best only able to use tiny torch pointed at ground, never towards Patient. During my most light sensitive phase, I had to don swimming goggles covered in tin foil to sleep past dawn in summer.	

COGNITIVE EFFECTS:	SEVERE ME PATIENTS	VERY SEVERE ME PATIENTS
Noise Sensitivity	Increased sensitivity to Noise common. Can last for months and in some cases, years. Pain as per very Severe Patients.	Patient extremely sensitive to Noise. Even the quiet whispers of a Carer can sound like a million decibels to the Patient. Feels like head is being pounded by a sledge hammer, and sometimes pain in head is just so excruciating, Patient feels like head is going to explode. Again, this symptom is linked to the dysfunction of the autonomic nervous system. Only way to cope is to reduce noise in/ex house and/or use ear plugs. But even ear plugs do not sometimes help, so noise-sensitive is Patient.
Sensitivity to Smell	Extremely sensitive to chemicals/ fragranced products/food smells. Coping strategies as per very Severe Patients.	Patient is hyper sensitive to smells and even the mere whiff of eg perfume/fabric conditioner on clothes/cooking smells can cause Severe bouts of nausea, headaches and/or migraines Carers/visitors/Patients all have to use unscented toiletries eg Green People No Scent range.

COGNITIVE EFFECTS:	SEVERE ME PATIENTS	VERY SEVERE ME PATIENTS
		Air purifiers can help, but only if Patient not sensitive to noise of machine.
Sensitivity to Touch	Yet another heart-breaking symptom of Severe M.E

At a time when Patient is absolutely terrified and so in need of a hug, many Patients are unable to be touched, even if only gently on the hand, let alone be hugged by loved ones. Even the gentlest of touches can cause Patients extreme pain, so sensitive are they to touch. | Some Patients extremely sensitive to touch. Even the lightest of touches on their bodies can result in extreme pain.

Only lightest of fabrics can be worn.

Bedding often has to be placed on a blanket frame so that Patient's body stays warm but is not touched by the covers. |
| Talking | Cognitive function severely impaired. Brain fog, memory loss, inability to process thoughts, cognitive confusion, inability to concentrate or follow conversation standard symptoms of Severe ME | Usually totally unable. |

COGNITIVE EFFECTS:	SEVERE ME PATIENTS	VERY SEVERE ME PATIENTS
Reading	Reading is really difficult for Severe Patients due to Severe cognitive dysfunction.

Even if Patient is out of the light sensitive phase, their brain simply cannot process the level of information coming in when they attempt to read anything; Patients can often see the words but not be able to clearly focus upon them, or make any sense of them. This is doubly terrifying as Patient worries that not only is their brain affected but also their eyesight.

When I progressed from very Severe to Severe ME, I could only look at a picture on a card for 5 seconds before my brain would | Totally unable. |

COGNITIVE EFFECTS:	SEVERE ME PATIENTS	VERY SEVERE ME PATIENTS
	begin to hurt; it would feel as if my head had been placed in a vice.	
	The following week, I would try to read one word, then two words the following week, then three words the week after etc, using pieces of cardboard that my Carers had made, to cover the text of a page that I was not ready to process.	
	Reading progress was frustratingly slow; but I had to re-train my brain to process the information coming into it from the pages in front of me, just as your loved one will have to do.	
	So, don't rush them, just support them and be thrilled for them when	

COGNITIVE EFFECTS:	SEVERE ME PATIENTS	VERY SEVERE ME PATIENTS
	you learn that they can read their first word.	
TV	TV is one of the most demanding activities for Patients as it stimulates the brain, eyes and ears simultaneously; if Patient is light sensitive then TV is totally impossible.

Severe ME Patients' cognitive function has been Severely affected by the illness and TV will be one of the hardest activities to rebuild into their life when they begin to recover.

If a Severely Affected Patient can tolerate any TV lying down, it is usually only for a few minutes egg once a week, followed by deep | Totally unable. |

COGNITIVE EFFECTS:	SEVERE ME PATIENTS	VERY SEVERE ME PATIENTS
	Rest period to calm down brain and nervous system.	
	If a Patient has not been able to watch TV for several weeks/ months, then Patient needs to start by watching the screen for eg 1 second, then switching it off; monitor the brain's reaction to TV's huge stimuli; then build up very very slowly over a period of months.	
	When I recovered from my light sensitive phase, I started first with listening to TV with eyes closed for 10 seconds; then the week after I watched the TV screen for 1 second, then the week after for 3 seconds; then the week after for 5 seconds...... you get the idea.	

COGNITIVE EFFECTS:	SEVERE ME PATIENTS	VERY SEVERE ME PATIENTS
	So, if you think your loved one is curled up in bed, watching a bit of TV to while away the time, think again!	
Radio	*May be able to listen to short bursts of gentle music/gentle talk, but as per TV, the speed at which Radio DJs talk may be just too fast for the Patients' brain to process.*	*Totally unable.*
Writing	*May be able to just about write their signature if Carer guides their hand, but nothing else; their hands/arms are just incapable of producing the energy and co-ordination and concentration needed to write.* *Patient will have to re-train their arm/hand muscles and re-build their levels of concentration to use*	*Totally unable.*

COGNITIVE EFFECTS:	SEVERE ME PATIENTS	VERY SEVERE ME PATIENTS
	a pen and write again once they move into the recovery phase. *When I started to tackle writing as part of my recovery programme, it took me 8 days to write THANK YOU on a piece of paper to my husband, mum and mum-in-law, writing 1 character per day*	
Email/Internet	*For Patients whose cognitive dysfunction is Severe, attempting to use a computer is usually impossible, as level of concentration required is too demanding.* *Likewise, if Patient is cognitively ready to attempt using a computer but is still light sensitive, then computer work is obviously out of the question.*	*Totally unable.*

I would also urge you to visit Claire Wade's website, www. survivingsevereme.com from which the following is a small excerpt:

"To me Severe ME is lying in a darkened room alone, trapped, frustrated and scared. Feeling things happen to your body that you can't stop or control: - the terrible headaches, muscle, joint and glandular pain, muscle spasms when your arms and legs jerk or even paralysis.

It is being awake all night with your brain in hyper-drive so you can't stop thinking. Feeling so exhausted you want to cry, but too tired to even do that."

Claire has also produced a fantastic booklet called 'Surviving Severe ME', available from www.survivingsevereme.com which I also strongly recommend.

Chapter 6: How long does Severe ME last?

The first thing you have to get your head around is that Severe ME is a long-haul illness; your relative or friend is not going to be physically disabled for a few days, a few weeks or a few months. Each Patient's experience is unique but you must realise that it may take years for your relative/friend to improve and you need to bear in mind that the life they lead will be dramatically different to the one they lived pre-Severe ME; and remember, setbacks and relapses will be part and parcel of a fluctuating illness like ME. Long term, Severe ME Patients can improve as can their quality of life, but only if they are given the right advice and the right support at the right time.

There seem to be three distinct phases in ME:

a.   Acute phase: Feels like body/brain in a kind of
                                              freefall.
                                              Energy levels deteriorate; normal
                                              function impossible.
                                              No control over what is happening to
                                              their body/brain.

b.   Chronic/plateau phase   Feels like world war III in body/brain.
                                              No progress made; plateaux usual.
                                              Terrifying time for Patient and Carer.
                                              May also be referred to as maintenance
                                              or stabilisation phase.

c.   Recovery phase   Body/brain starts to self-correct if given
                                              right advice/treatment at right time.
                                              Improvement begins.
                                              Setbacks/Relapses part of recovery
                                              phase.

Sadly, setbacks and/or relapses are part and parcel of the recovery process for many Patients but you can really help the Carer and the Patient by helping them try to identify the causes/triggers of the setback and put together a plan to avoid them in the future.

Chapter 7: How is Severe ME treated and managed?

Many factors contribute to contracting Severe ME. Likewise, many factors contribute to a Patient's chances of improving; but you must always remember that each Patient is unique – what works for one Severe ME Patient may or may not work for another and indeed what does not work for a Patient at one stage in their recovery, may then work well for them at another stage of their recovery from this bewildering illness.

So, it would be totally irresponsible of me to simply lay out a step-by-step plan as to how I escaped the living hell of Severe ME.

Each Patient's experience of Severe ME is unique to them, and until a comprehensive diagnostic test and corresponding curative treatment protocol is discovered, what I need to do is to point you in the direction of those organisations/individuals/teams/sources of expert information that can help you, the Carer and the rest of the Patient's family/friends piece together the recovery jigsaw for **your** loved one; I will also attempt to give you an overview of treatments/management techniques that you will no doubt come across in your research together with my thoughts of them.

1. Sources of Information

Listed below are the sources of information that I have found extremely useful, and so wish that someone had told my family/ friends and I about at the **start** of my illness. You will also find on Page 104 a list of Books that proved very useful in my recovery.

Action for ME - www.actionforme.org.uk

Action for ME is a leading charity for people with ME and their Carers.

Action For ME, 42 Temple Street, Keynsham BS31 1EH
Telephone: 0117 927 9551
Email: questions@actionforme.org.uk

They have a section entitled *Find Local Services* where you can enter your postcode to find specialist services are in your area.

The ME Association - www.meassociation.org.uk

Leading ME Charity dedicated to informing and supporting those affected by ME.

They have compiled a brilliant list of **NHS Specialist Services round the UK** available to ME patients on their website http://www.meassociation.org.uk/nhsspecialistservices/
If you have trouble with this link, the list can be found at the end of their **Helpful Services** Section on their website under **Quick Links** or telephone them for details on 0844 576 5326 (times as below).
(See Appendix 1 at back of this Info Pack for print out of ME Association's NHS Specialist Services around the UK)

ME Connect is the telephone and email helpline service of The ME Association. It provides support for people with ME and those who live with or care for them.
Telephone 0844 576 5326 (10am-12pm, 2-4pm, 7-9pm)

Email: meconnect@meassociation.org.uk

25% ME Group - www.25megroup.org

The 25% ME Group exists to focus on Severe ME and support all who have the severe form of ME and those who care for them.

The 25% ME Group, 21 Church Street, Troon, Ayrshire KA10 6HT
Telephone: 01292 318611 (9.30am-5pm Mon-Fri)
Email: enquiry@25megroup.org

Surviving Severe ME – www.survivingsevereme.com

Website set up by Claire Wade who understands Severe ME first hand, having become ill at the age of 10 and bedbound for 6 years, in a darkened room 24/7. The website is full of practical, useful information to sufferers and carers alike, specifically about Severe ME.

Severe ME – A Guide to Living by Emily Collingridge

A comprehensive book for patients with Severe ME and the loved ones and professionals caring for them is now available from www.severeme.info

To order a copy go online to www.severeme.info

The Young ME Sufferers Trust – www.tymestrust.org

Tymes Trust is an established national UK service for children and young people with ME and their families.

Tymes Trust, PO Box 4347, Stock, Ingatestone, CM4 9TE
Telephone 0845 003 9002
Email via their contact form on website

Dr Sarah Myhill – www.drmyhill.co.uk

A highly informative website by Dr Sarah Myhill, a specialist in ME. She has also produced a book entitled *Diagnosis & Treatment of CFS/ME* which can be purchased from her website.

Dr Sarah Myhill, Upper Weston, Llangunllo, Knighton, Powys, LD7 ISL
Telephone 01547 550 331

Dr Myhill has also set up a very useful online shop selling supplements recommended in her treatment protocol. www.salesatdrmyhill.co.uk

Email: sales@doctormyhill.co.uk

CFS Service, Essex Neurosciences Unit, Barking, Havering and Redbridge NHS Trust

Sadly, Professor Findley's renowned in-patient CFS Service (which I was extremely fortunate to be admitted to during my illness) which developed into a national referral centre, with a special expertise in the assessment and management of those patients with severe and very severe fatigue syndromes, has been closed. There is a weekly NHS outpatient clinic at the Queens Hospital, Romford, Essex currently run by Dr A Chaudhuri (telephone 01708 504147 for details)

You Wellbeing – www.youwellbeing.com

Co-founded by Sarah Marshall (herself a recovered ME patient) and Ashley Meyer, London based You Wellbeing clinic has been working within the specialist field of ME, CFS, PVFS, CFIDS and Fibromyalgia for almost 20 years. **They are happy to offer consultation via telephone/skype/ facetime for patients and carers unable to travel to London**. They offer a free information report as well as a free initial chat with a practitioner.

Telephone 020 8371 8202
Email hello@youwellbeing.com

The Optimum Health Clinic – www.theoptimumhealthclincic.com

Set up by Alex Howard, (himself a recovered ME patient), is an integrative private medical clinic with a specialism in the diagnosis and treatment of ME, CFS and Fibromyalgia along with complementary and alternative medicine-based approaches for optimising health, relaxation and general wellbeing.

They are happy to offer consultation via telephone/skype/ facetime for patients and their carers unable to travel.

They offer a free information pack as well as a free 15-minute initial chat with a practitioner.

The Optimum Health Clinic, Bickerton House, 25-27 Bickerton Road, London N19 5JT
Telephone 0845 226 1762

The Hummingbirds' Foundation for ME – www.hfme.org

Fighting for recognition of ME and for patients to be accorded the same basic human rights as those with similar devastating neurological diseases such as MS. A good source of information.

ME Research UK – www.meresearch.org.uk

ME Research UK is a charity which exists to fund biomedical research into ME/CFS, to find its cause, to develop effective treatments and ultimately to discover a cure.

ME Research UK, The Gateway, North Methven Street, Perth PH1 5PP
Telephone 01738 451234
Email meruk@pkavs.org.uk
Facebook www.facebook.com/MEResearchUK

2. Overview of treatments

As you will know by now, Severe ME has a huge variety of symptoms that need to be managed – there is no single magic cure-all-pill yet, but there are several therapeutic strategies that can make a difference to Patients and help them control their symptoms, so aiding the improvement:

It will help you enormously in your research if you have an overview of 'tools' that the Patient may use to aid their improvement, and a basic understanding of the terminology that you might come across:

2.1 <u>Energy Management</u>:

Sometimes also referred to as *Activity Management*. I prefer to call it *Energy Management* because that is exactly what Patients have to learn to do – just as Diabetics have to learn to manage their sugar levels, so ME Patients have to learn to manage their energy levels. The aim is to plan activities with military precision to avoid the peaks and troughs so often experienced by Patients, in effect to establish a consistent and sustainable level of daily activity that avoids relapses through over exertion, usually referred to as 'Baselines'.

For example, say a Severe ME Patient is ready to attempt to feed themselves; if they have been being fed by their Carer lying down, to attempt to sit up and lift the spoon to their mouths say 20 times with the right arm in one huge leap forward, well that would simply exhaust the Patient and lead to a major trough/setback afterwards, heavy aching muscles, exhaustion, anxiety etc; **but** if the activity was planned out in tiny manageable steps...

eg with the Patient first of all sitting up for 10 seconds for 5 days, then 20 seconds for the next 5 days, then 30 seconds for the next 5 days, then 45 seconds for 5 days, then 1 minute for 5 days, then 2 minutes for 5 days, aiming in the end to be able to sit up in bed for say 5 minutes without a major flare up of symptoms; and then the lifting of the spoon to the mouth incorporated into the activity, say lifting 1 spoonful of food with the right arm, then 1 spoonful with the left arm for 5 days, then 2 spoonful's each arm for the next 5 days, then 3 spoonful's each arm for the next 5 days, building up to say 20 spoonfuls each arms...

... well, then increasing the activity would have been managed very carefully and built up very slowly, hopefully preventing the

Patient from experiencing a very frightening trough or bad flare up of symptoms.

When you read about Energy *Management/Activity Management* you will probably also come across other phrases such as the following: *Rest & Deep Relaxation techniques, Pacing, Graded Activity/Rest Programmes and Switching.*

And it is my firm belief that *Energy Management* incorporating *Rest & Deep Relaxation techniques, Pacing, Graded Activity/ Rest Programmes and Switching* is the single most important treatment 'area' for all Severe ME Patients, whatever stage of the illness they are at, whatever the severity of their symptoms.

So, let's look at them one by one.

a)   Rest & Deep Relaxation Techniques

Learning what true Rest means is probably one of the most important lessons that Patients need to learn.
In chapter 3 I explained that a Severe ME Patient is 'stuck' in the stressful 'fight or flight' state **almost permanently**; their primary body systems are greatly affected: breathing, muscles/joints, blood circulation, special senses, digestion, whilst their brain is working overtime constantly in a problem-solving manner – utterly and completely exhausting. So, it is vital that Patients find a way of calming down their Sympathetic Nervous System.

When I use the term 'Rest' in relation to treatments for Severe ME, it really means 'Deep Relaxation'. Resting is not reading a book, watching TV or even quietly daydreaming. A period of Deep Relaxation, true rest, is a period of quiet time, lying down, when the Patient aims to reduce down all stimulation of their senses, thereby allowing the body to rest, heal and start to self-correct. Basically, the Patient needs to learn how to quieten the body and the brain, not easy, but as I have said vital.

Indeed, when I was at my most Severe, bed-bound, light sensitive, in constant pain, sleeping perhaps 3-4 hours a night if I was lucky, unable to do anything for myself, lying in my bed awake, anxious, and terrified at what was happening to me for 20 hours a day was anything but restful…but when I was taught by Professor Findley's CFS/ME team how to switch off my racing brain and calm down my Sympathetic Nervous System, well, the difference to my life and the speed at which my improvement picked up was nothing short of amazing.

How to Relax:

Creating a feeling of relaxation incorporates being able to switch off both physically and mentally. There are a number of strategies the Patient can use to help them achieve this:

i)   Breathing Exercises
ii) Listening to soft instrumental relaxation music
iii) Following a guided relaxation technique.

Listed below are good sources of information and/or suppliers of CDs/tapes that could be of benefit to your loved on:

New World Music Ltd - www.newworldmusic.com
Suppliers of wide range of guided relaxation CDs, relaxing music CDs and other relaxation related products.
New World Music, Harmony House, Hillside Road East, Bungay, Suffolk NR35 1RX
Telephone: 01986 891 600

Angela Stevens – www.angela-stevens.co.uk
Breathe to Live CD is specifically for people with Severe ME as the breathing exercises can be practised if bedbound.
Telephone: 01892 782 865
Email: info@angela-stevens.co.

Breathworks – www.breathworks-mindfulness.co.uk
Telephone: 0203 856 9561 or 0161 834 1110
Email: info@breathworks.co.uk
An organisation whose breathing exercises and meditations can be done if bedbound

Audio Meditation: www.audiomeditation.co.uk

Downloadable meditations available
Telephone: 020 3286 6478
Email: info@augiomeditation.co.uk

I would also like to cover the area of Autogenic Relaxation, an area which I found to be one of the most powerful forms of Deep Relaxation, so I have outlined below a basic Autogenic exercise, maybe you could perhaps record onto tape/CD for your loved one, or take a copy and give it to his/her Carer to read out to them:

Autogenic Relaxation (Patient listening to Carer version)

Lying down get as comfortable and supported as you can – use pillows under your arms/legs if you need to – then close your eyes and imagine that your arms and legs feel heavy. Don't try too hard, just be aware of your arms and legs, then listen to me as I repeat some phrases to you, and feel your arms and legs feeling relaxed and heavy as we work through this relaxation:

My right arm is heavy, my right arm is heavy, my right arm is heavy

My left arm is heavy, my left arm is heavy, my left arm is heavy

My right leg is heavy, my right leg is heavy, my right leg is heavy

My left leg is heavy, my left leg is heavy, my left leg is heavy

My arms and legs are heavy, my arms and legs are heavy, my arms and legs are heavy

I am relaxed and at peace (PAUSE)

My neck and shoulders are relaxed and heavy

I am relaxed and at peace (PAUSE)

*Now imagine that your arms and legs feel heavy **and** warm; feel the warmth flowing down through your arms from your shoulder, down your arms into your fingers and down your legs into your feet and toes, and again listen to me as I talk you through this relaxation:*

My right arm is heavy and warm, my right arm is heavy and warm, my right arm is heavy and warm

My left arm is heavy and warm, my left arm is heavy and warm, my left arm is heavy and warm

My right leg is heavy and warm, my right leg is heavy and warm, my right leg is heavy and warm

My left leg is heavy and warm, my left leg is heavy and warm, my left leg is heavy and warm

My arms and legs are heavy, my arms and legs are heavy, my arms and legs are heavy

I am relaxed and at peace (PAUSE)

My neck and shoulders are relaxed and heavy

I am relaxed and at peace (PAUSE)

My breathing is slow relaxed and even

My heart beat is calm and regular

My stomach is calm and warm

My forehead is cool and clear

I am relaxed and at peace

Now just lay there and enjoy this feeling of complete relaxation for a few minutes (PAUSE)

Ok, now it is time to finish, but know that when you open your eyes, you will feel very relaxed and carry this sense of peace with you throughout the coming days.

As you can see, Autogenic Relaxation is pretty straightforward, the main objective being to rest both the mind and body; but if it is simply too much for the Patient to listen to a tape of this relaxation or someone reading it out to them very, very slowly, then the Patient could try to just say a few of the phrases over to themselves in their heads, to quieten the brain's 'chatter', eg

my arms and legs are relaxed, heavy and warm (Pause)

I am relaxed and at peace (Pause)

My arms and legs are relaxed, heavy and warm (Pause)

I am relaxed and at peace (Pause)

(Repeat over and over....)

Alternatively, if they are at the stage of the illness when their brain is just too foggy then they could try doing something else; when I was just too ill to do a full autogenic relaxation, I would simply lay still, close my eyes, put in my earplugs and just say to myself over and over again a simple relaxing mantra like 'relax', 'calm', 'heal' or 'peace', in my head, which proved just as relaxing and calming. I would be lying down, trying to become aware of my breathing, inhaling slowly, and exhaling slowly, on the outward breath, I would just say to myself *'and Re-Lax...'*, and just keep repeating for about 10 minutes, before listening to some very soothing, gentle relaxation music for the rest of my 30minute rest period.

Like all things learning to relax takes practice, as the racing brain keeps wanting to break into the Patients' thoughts, but if they stick with it and keep trying, they will find that it becomes easier, and easier.

Indeed, when I talk to people about Rest and Relaxation periods, I tell them that I regard my 30-minute Rest Periods in just the same way as I would a Prescription for a medicine, because for Severe ME Patients that is precisely what they are, a prescription for an effective treatment that will aid recovery.

b) **<u>Pacing</u>**

To improve, the Patient has to learn to manage successfully activity alongside rest to establish a consistent and sustainable level of daily activity that avoids relapses through over exertion – this is called *pacing.*

Action for ME has a downloadable booklet on Pacing and how it can help Patients. Called *'Pacing for people with ME'* it is available from www.actionforme.org.uk but do bear in mind that the booklet has been written for all grades of ME, including Mild and Moderate, but it does explain the concept of Pacing well.
Telephone: 0117 927 9551
Email: questions@actionforme.org.uk

Learning to pace can help the Patient start to take control of their condition and enable them to become an expert in managing their condition. However, whilst 'Pacing Yourself' when you are ill might sound a lot like common sense, that does **not** mean that it is easy. I would say that it is one of the single most difficult things that I had to learn during my illness, and the discipline required is unimaginable, but it works. So, getting hold of a copy of this booklet for the Carer would be an enormous help as they can then work steadily with the Patient to put it into practice.

c)   **Graded Activity/Rest Programmes and Switching**

So now that we have looked at Deep Relaxation/Rest techniques and Pacing individually, let's look at how the Patient needs to put them into practice.

There a couple of key points here. Before a Patient can even attempt to pace themselves, they need to be made aware that **three types of energy** are involved in all their daily activities:

Physical Energy (eg lying, sitting, eating, standing, walking)
Mental or Cognitive Energy (eg thinking, reading, TV, radio)
Emotional (eg happy, sad, anxious, angry)

And some activities require all three types of energy eg talking to a close friend/relative that the Patient has been unable to see for several months – the physical energy required to actually talk, the mental energy required to concentrate and formulate sentences, and the emotional energy of seeing a loved one that the Patient has so missed.

Then there is the need to **grade each activity into a low energy, a medium energy or a high energy activity.** For example, for a Severely affected ME Patient talking to their Carer for 2 minutes might be graded as a medium energy activity, but talking to medical specialist on a home visit for 2 minutes, whom they have never met before, well, that would probably be graded as a very high energy activity, because there would probably be a high level of anxiety involved.

Another clever technique to help Patients manage their precious energy is that of **Switching.** When I started to improve, I found that if I kept switching between different activities, ie using different parts of the brain and different muscle groups, then I could actually do more over the

course of a day. This concept is very well explained in a book **'Somebody Help ME – Self Help Guide for ME Sufferers and their Families'** by Jill Moss, which is available from www. amazon.co.uk

To give you an idea of what an Activity/Rest Programme can look like, below is a copy of my Programme when I was about one year into my recovery phase:

TIME	ACTIVITY	ENERGY GRADE (low/ medium/ high)
7.45-8am	*Wake up and come to*	*Low*
8-9.30am	*Carer sort bedroom out, give me breakfast and 5 min chat. Feed self and take vitamins (all lying down on bed)*	*Medium*
	Listen Radio News, stretches lying down.	*Medium*

	Wall 8 paces loo, wash at sink sitting on perch stool.	*High*
9.30-10am	*R E S T*	
10-11am	*Get dressed sitting on bed and put moisturizer on face.*	*High*
	Listen Classical Music (lying down on bed)	*Low*
	Sit out for 5 mins in bedroom chair, high backed, to write (4 paces to chair, hand on wall as walk to maintain balance)	*Medium*
11-11.30am	*R E S T*	
11.30-12.30	*Walk 8 paces loo, and then another 4 paces into spare bedroom overlooking back garden.*	*Medium*
	Flick through easy (mainly pictures) magazines (5 minutes) lying on day bed.	*Low*
	Carer brings lunch, 5 min chat; can feed self lying on day bed.	*Medium*
12.30-1pm	*R E S T*	
1-2pm	*Walk 4 paces loo, walk back over wooden step block (starting to re train muscles in preparation for tackling 2 steps needed to get on/off newly installed Stairlift)*	*High*
	Ly on front on day bed, listen Classic FM	*Low*

	Ly on back, read magazine or 5 min telephone call or listen radio.	*Medium*
2-2.30pm	*R E S T*	
2.30-3.30pm	*Therapist/Visitor or telephone call (lying on bed)*	*High*
	Light music lying	*Low*
	Afternoon snack, feed self lying	*Low*
3.30-4pm	*R E S T*	
4-5.30pm	*Walk loo, then sit in high backed chair 5 mins.*	*Medium*
	Walk 100 paces between landing/ bedrooms.	*High*
	Lying, watch TV 10 minutes	*Medium*
5.15-5.45pm	*R E S T*	
5.45-6.45pm	*Walk loo, walk back over wooden step block*	*Medium*
	Carer brings, Dinner, feed self lying quiet	*Medium*
	Magazine read	*Medium*
	Chat 10 minutes to Carer or telephone call 5 minutes	*High*
6.45-7.15pm	*R E S T*	

7.15-8.30pm	*Walk loo, wash at sink, sitting on perch stool*	*High*
		Low
	Listen classic FM, lying	*High*
	Supper and 5-minute chat with	*Low*
	Carer, or back massage from Carer.	*Medium*
	Listen Classic FM, lying	
	Brush Teeth (using bowl brought by Carer at Dinner), undress sitting up on bed.	
8,30-9pm	*WIND DOWN RELAXATION TAPE*	
9pm	*Sleep*	

2.2 Cognitive Behaviour Therapy (CBT) & Graded Exercise Therapy (GET)

Cognitive Behaviour Therapy (CBT) was developed in the 1950s and is a psychological treatment that looks at how a person's thoughts, beliefs, behaviour and physical symptoms all fit together.

Debate rages on as to whether CBT is a suitable therapy for ME Patients, Radio 4 broadcast a series of programmes about ME (for full transcripts go to www.bbc.co.uk/radio4/youandyours/ me_series.shtml), with the first programme focusing on CBT. Dr Charles Shepherd of the ME Association was one of the Speakers, and I think he pretty much says it all for me:

"CBT seems to be moving into all kinds of illnesses…and this is perhaps the argument that NICE would make – that it's used sometimes with the management of Cancer and serious physical illnesses like Multiple Sclerosis. But I think this argument is disingenuous. (CBT) is not a primary form of treatment there, as is being recommended for people with ME. If you went along to a Cancer Specialist and were just offered CBT as the primary

form of treatment you'd be quite horrified, in fact you'd probably think you were being treated with medical negligence"

Even when we consider CBT as a <u>supporting</u> treatment for ME Patients, it is important that you, the Severe ME Patient's family and friends, bear in mind that any clinical studies that claim that CBT and GET can improve the functional capacity of ME Patients have focused on *ambulant adult ME Patients.* **The key fact to remember here, is that these studies have focused on Mildly Affected Patients, and NOT Severe ME Patients, a fact that many non-specialist medical professionals conveniently choose to ignore.**

I have had three experiences of CBT – two terrible, one excellent. CBT that focuses purely on the need for positive thinking is a highly dangerous therapy to all levels of ME Patients. I know. Over positive encouragement from a Psychologist specialising in CBT, pushing me to return to work in 1998 catapulted me from Mild ME into the horrors of Very Severe ME; and again in 2000 another CBT specialist pushed me too far too fast causing me a terrible relapse, wasting another year of my life.

However, my other experience of CBT was excellent - yes, Severe ME Patients have to be positive, but they must always **balance that positivity with caution**. Highly experienced medical professionals who worked with Severe ME Patients, day in day out, focused on the need for **accurate thinking**; calm, rational thinking not purely over pushy, positive thinking that is so very dangerous to Severe ME Patients. It is this type of therapy that I believe **can** help Severe ME Patients but it is vital that any medical professional has a lot of experience of working with Severe ME Patients, not just Mildly or Moderately affected, so make sure that you stress this point to the Carer if any medical professional is recommending CBT for your loved one.

Now onto **Graded Exercise Therapy (GET),** and I want you to read the opinion of Professor Findley, Neurologist and head of the National ME Centre, as published in a great article on GET in AFME's (www.afme.org.uk) Interaction Magazine in December 2006:

".... As regards GET, this concept is based on very limited clinical evidence. The two major trials which are quoted only looked at ambulant Patients who were Mild to Moderate in terms of severity. There is no information on GET in Patients who are Severely or very Severely affected.

Clinical experience has demonstrated that some Patients may be made worse with GET, particularly if it is unsupervised and not carefully monitored.
Those of us who are looking after Severe and very Severe Patients can confirm that in this group, GET will result in relapse and deterioration.

The approach to rehabilitation in this group must be through careful management of all the perpetuating factors of the fatigue state, eg sleep disturbance, pain, mood, anxiety, allergy, food intolerances etc as part of a holistic programme, including carefully structured and monitored activities of daily living in a graduated fashion, preferably under the supervision of a multi-disciplinary fatigue team.

GET has a place in those Patients who are able to sustain a whole day's activity and can use simple exercise, proceeding from sub-anaerobic levels to aerobic levels over time. Clearly if any exercise results in a significant deterioration in functioning, or increase in symptoms, ie that is not just transient, then the whole programme needs to be revised.

Careful, Mild, incremental exercise will help with de-conditioning and improve stamina in mobile, Mild to Moderate Patients, or in those who have improved to that level of functioning.

In the studies carried out so far, GET has never been used in isolation (this would be impossible to do). It has always been part of a therapeutic regime, including advice on symptom management and lifestyle changes.

If you have concerns about the possible adverse effects of GET, then you should seek the advice of a CFS specialist to ascertain whether in your case it would be reasonable to try GET in a supervised manner.

The attraction of any health authority to recommend GET is that it is cheap and ostensibly easy to apply. However, this ignores the fact that CFS/ME does not equate to lack of fitness, but is a complex disorder of the nervous system and its connection with the immune system."

Professor Findley headed up the CFS service based at Queens Hospital, Romford, Essex, one of the very few UK centres to admit Severely affected CFS/ME Patients for in-patient care and I was one of the lucky few that benefited from his expertise. Sadly, Professor Findley has now retired but his treatment protocol is still followed by some clinics, and rightly so.

2.3 Nutritional Therapy

There is much anecdotal evidence that dietary changes coupled with nutritional supplements help many Severe ME Patients, myself included. If you want to research this area then the contacts listed below may be a good place to start:

Dr Sarah Myhill – www.drmyhill.co.uk

A highly informative website by Dr Sarah Myhill, a specialist in ME. She has also produced a book entitled *Diagnosis & Treatment of CFS/ME* which can be purchased from her website.

Dr Sarah Myhill, Upper Weston, Llangunllo, Knighton, Powys, LD7 ISL
Telephone 01547 550 331

Dr Myhill has also set up a very useful online shop selling supplements recommended in her treatment protocol. www. salesatdrmyhill.co.uk
Email: sales@doctormyhill.co.uk

You Wellbeing – www.youwellbeing.com

Co-founded by Sarah Marshall (herself a recovered ME patient) and Ashley Meyer, London based You Wellbeing clinic has been working within the specialist field of ME, CFS, PVFS, CFIDS and Fibromyalgia for almost 20 years. **They are happy to offer consultation via telephone/skype/ facetime for patients and carers unable to travel to London**. They offer a free information report as well as a free initial chat with a practitioner. They often work alongside a specialist Nutritional Therapist.

Telephone 020 8371 8202
Email hello@youwellbeing.com

The Optimum Health Clinic – www.theoptimumhealthclincic. com

Set up by Alex Howard, (himself a recovered ME patient), is an integrative private medical clinic with a specialism in the diagnosis and treatment of ME, CFS and Fibromyalgia along with complementary and alternative medicine-based approaches for optimising health, relaxation and general wellbeing. **They are happy to offer consultation via telephone/skype/facetime for patients and their carers unable to travel.** They offer a free information pack as well as a free 15-minute initial chat with a practitioner and work often alongside specialist Nutritional Therapists.

The Optimum Health Clinic, Bickerton House, 25-27 Bickerton Road, London N19 5JT
Telephone 0845 226 1762

Pro Health – www.ImmuneSupport.com

American based company set up to provide active support of CFS and Fibromyalgia research and advocacy. Very good on-line information library and on-line mail order shop for nutritional supplements designed for CFS/ME Patients. Happy to post their products worldwide.

Pro Health also has a great link to the well-known Dr Teitelbaum's Protocol for CFS & Fibromyalgia - www. immunesupport.com/chronic-fatigue-syndrome-teitelbaum.htm

Leading suppliers of supplements with in house, trained, nutritionists who can offer advice.

BioCare Ltd – www.biocare.co.uk

Lakeside, 180 Lifford Lane, Kings Norton, Birmingham B30 3NU
Telephone 0121 433 3727 Sales & General Enquiries
Telephone 0121 433 8702 Technical Support (Nutritionist)

Solgar Vitamin and Herb Company (UK) – www.solgar.com

Adbury, Tring, Herts HP23 5PT
Telephone 01442 890355

Kudos Vitamins and Herbal – www.kudosvitamins.com

2nd Floor, Parkway House, Sheen Lane, East Sheen, London SW14 8LS
Telephone 020 8392 6524

The NutriCentre – www.nutricentre.com

The Hale Clinic, 7 Park Crescent, London W1N 3HE
Telephone 020 7436 0422

Viridian Nutrition Ltd – www.viridian-nutrition.com

31 Alvis Way, Daventry, Northants NN11 5PG
Telephone 01327 878050

Igennus – www.vegepa.com

Telephone 0845 1300424

www.thevegaepaformescheme.com is also worth checking out for discounted Vegepa, which may be helpful in treating the symptoms of Severe ME

Also remember the CFS/ME NHS Helpline which is, at time of writing, being piloted for the South West/Greater Manchester:

2.4 Sleep, Pain and Mood Problems

It is worth remembering that with any illness there will be a degree of associated mood problems, whether they manifest as anxiety, depression, despair, irritability or mood swings; and for Patients with Severe ME, an illness that is so terribly disabling and utterly bewildering, and understood by so few medical professionals... well, it would be odd if the Patient didn't experience some kind of mood problem, wouldn't it?

I suffered badly with panic attacks, anxiety and depression – shut away in a darkened room for best part of 18 months, unable to walk, talk, in constant pain, unable to do anything for myself and with little medical support or help for so long – and that meant that throughout my recovery journey I had to constantly fight those feelings of panic and terror of returning to those dark days, so if your friend/relative finds him/herself in a similar situation, and is offered anti-depressant medication by their GP to help them through, then do have the utmost compassion and understanding of what they are enduring and remember, that like the other symptoms, these secondary emotions will pass too, but that in the meantime that medication may be just what they need to keep their spirits up to fight on.

One vital point to bear in mind if you do find yourself discussing the subject of sleep/pain/mood medication with the Carer/Patient, is that Severe ME Patients are highly sensitive to many drugs; so, if the Patient does try any new medication, it is wise to start at a greatly reduced dosage. When I started Amitriptyline (tricyclic antidepressant which controlled my pain, improved my sleep, cleared brain fog and eased anxiety attacks) I started at ½ mg per day – a normal person's starting dose is 75mgs.

2.5 Complementary Medicine

Many Severe ME Patients, myself included, turn to complementary treatments when faced with how little conventional medicine can offer us at the present time.

So outlined below is some information which might give you a start point for investigating complementary therapies for your friend/relative; as I have said before, each Patient is unique, what works for one Severe ME Patient may or may not work for another, **so approach with caution**, and if I had to give just one piece of advice which I wish someone had given to me it would be this: your first question should always be *'How much experience do you have of treating Severe and Very Severe ME Patients and do you have any testimonials from them?'*. **Unless they can answer this question positively, then steer well clear.**

The Complementary Medical Association www.the-cma.org. uk

Telephone: 0845 129 8434

Institute can give you advice about specific alternative therapies and put you in touch with practitioners and societies.

Chapter 8: How can Family and Friends help?

I cannot stress enough just how much difference your support can make to a Patient's chances of improving. My husband and I were incredibly lucky to have the support of so many of our relatives and friends, without whom, my recovery would not have been possible.

If **you** want to help someone with Severe ME, there are three precious gifts you can give to them and their Carer(s):

- **UNDERSTANDING**
- **CONSTANCY**
- **UNCONDITIONAL SUPPORT**

1. Understanding

Having a disabling illness is hard enough but having a disabling illness which is still often surrounded by ignorance and scepticism, is a nightmare. **You** can help to change this.

Severe ME Patients and their Carers simply do not have the energy or time to expend on constantly having to convince 'Doubting Thomas's that this is a serious physical illness. So, this is where you come in; you need to take responsibility for your own understanding of this illness, and that of those closest to you. Here's how:

1.1 Learn

Join National ME Charities such as Action For ME, The ME Association and The 25% ME Group; get on their websites, read their magazines, read the recommended books; learn all you can about Severe ME – the more informed you are, the more you will understand what your loved one is going through. (See Chapter 7 and Chapter 11 for contact details)

1.2 Listen

But, remember, each Patient's experience of Severe ME is unique; each Patient's symptoms and their recovery can vary dramatically; what works for one Patient that you read/hear about may or may not work for your loved one, or it may be that it will only work in a particular phase of their illness; and remember treatments that work so well for those Mildly or Moderately affected may **not** work for those Severely affected. It is this aspect of Severe ME that is so bewildering and so very frustrating.

So, you need to really listen to the Carer(s)/ Patient, really get to grips with all their individual symptoms, and if you are struggling to understand, **ask, ask, ask.**

The Patient will have little energy and will often be unable to talk for more than a few seconds/minutes if at all, but their Carer(s) witness every aspect of the nightmare with them, they become experts themselves, so ask them; Carers will always make time to explain the details of the illness to those people who are clearly making a huge effort to understand and help out.

1.3 Educate Others

Remember that everyone else is likely to be on the same steep learning curve as yourself, so whatever knowledge, research, facts you learn, **share** that information with relatives and friends who perhaps are not as proactive as you.

And if you come across Doubting Thomas', bombard them with information, send them copies of articles you come across, follow them up with a phone call/email to make sure they have understood, make them join the National ME Charities, in short, do not let them off the hook.

Sadly, I had a small number of relatives and friends who were Doubting Thomas's, and the stress they caused my husband and I was huge; so, if you can educate others like them and save your loved one from enduring such hurtful disbelief, you will be helping them enormously.

2.   <u>Constancy</u>

Severe ME is a long-haul illness.

It is not an illness where you can pop a few get well cards in the post, get on with your life and know that the Patient will be up and around again soon.

When Severely Affected Patients first become bed-bound, they and their Carers are usually inundated by cards, letters, flowers, calls, gifts and offers of help from well-wishers; but as the weeks roll into months and the months roll into years, for many Patients/ Carers, that early flow of support which gave them so much strength, largely starts to dry up and they struggle to understand how some relatives and friends could have abandoned them.

But when you start to look at the situation from the friends and family's perspective, you can perhaps see their conundrum. Knowing from the Carer(s) that the Patient is lying in a darkened bedroom, in terrible pain, too ill to feed themselves or walk to the loo, let alone talk on the telephone, read, write, or receive visitors, they simply cannot see how it would help the Patient if they were to continue sending cards/letters/flowers/gifts or asking if they can visit/call. So, friends and family simply get on with their daily lives, continuing to think about their loved one but not knowing what else to do. <u>But I firmly believe that this is a total cop-out.</u>

One thing you have to remember - Severe ME Patients and their Carer(s) are NOT TELEPATHIC. It's all very well thinking about the Patient and hoping and praying that they get better, but if you don't tell them that, how the hell are they

supposed to know or take comfort and strength from your concern.

And there is loads that you can do to help the Patient and their Carer(s), you just have to think outside the box, as some of our friends and family did; and over the next few pages I am going to outline some ways that you can help, ways that will show that you think about them all the time, that you would do anything to stop their pain and suffering, that you miss them terribly and would do anything to help them recover and get their lives back.

But make no mistake, if you do want to support your loved one through this bewildering illness, then you have to decide here and now whether you have the staying power to stand by them and their Carer(s) for as long as their recovery journey takes. If you are not in it for the long haul then bow out now and save them the sense of loss farther down the line.

3.   Support

3.1 Unconditional Support

Before they fell ill, Severe ME Patients are likely to have fulfilled numerous roles: daughter/son, wife/husband, mother/father, close friend, sister/brother, colleague/ boss, fellow student, school friend, team mate, neighbour, confidante etc.

ME Patients are often real 'givers' when they were well – a shoulder to lean on; a voice on the end of the phone to share in your joys, to listen to your problems; someone to turn to for advice, help, guidance; someone to lend a hand and offer practical support whenever you needed it, someone you could rely on to always be there. Well, because of this terrible illness, they cannot be there for you as they once were; they cannot fulfil their previous roles, and that is something you will have to come to terms with, and fast.

For the duration of their illness, the Severely affected ME Patient has absolutely nothing to give to you, which means that their virtual 'disappearance' from your life will be a huge loss, and your sadness, grief and frustration will be immense. But this is not about you; this is not about your loss, this is not about your grief; this is about them. This is where you have to put their needs and those of their Carers' first – they have nothing to give, so your support, in whatever form it takes, must be 100% unconditional.

3.2 What kind of supporter are you?

When you are considering how to help out, first of all, ask yourselves a few pertinent questions?

Do you live locally?
Do you drive?
Do you have a lot of free time?
How organised are you?
Are you forgetful?
Do you have any experience of dealing with long term illness?
Have you ever nursed a sick person?
Are you a calm person?
Are you reliable?
Do you have staying power?
Do you have cash to spare?
If you promise to do something, will you?
Are you a sensitive person?
Are you open minded?
Are you someone who is happy to roll your sleeves up and get stuck in, to whatever needs doing?
Are you happier surfing the internet for helpful research, than being near a sick person?
Could you become a campaigner?

The above questions are designed to start you thinking about what kind of person you are, and how you could best help. On the next page I have jotted down some loose categories of supporter types – **what kind would you like to be? Or, perhaps more importantly, what kind of supporter do you not want to be?**

The Good:

Rocks Often the main Carer, eg a partner or parent.
Their faith in the Patient never falters.
Strong, solid, 100% supportive.
Helping the Patient recover becomes their sole focus in life.
Source of immense strength to Patient.

Oaks Often a close relative/friend.
Always there for Patient/Carer to lean upon.
Very good at thinking outside the box and finding ways to support both Patient and
Carer, practically and emotionally, even if far away.
In it for the long haul, whatever happens.
Source of great strength and comfort to both Patient and Carer.

Bricks Friends or relatives, constant in their support, but at a lower level than Oaks.
Quick learners who really listen, learn and understand and whose support is constant.
Believe in Patient and Carer 100%.
These guys are bad time friends as well as good time friends.
Quick to volunteer, help and make sure Patient/ Carer knows they are there for them and thinking of them, constantly.
Real source of strength and help to Patient/Carer.

JIBs   Short for 'Jack in the boxes'.

People who really surprise the Patient/Carer with their proactive support.

Often friends/relatives who are not that close or had 'dropped' out of their lives, but hearing of the situation, rally round and offer ongoing practical and emotional support, often from afar.

Source of strength to Patient/Carer.

The Bad:

Butterflies   These people mean well and do care, but just do not want to become too involved.

They flit in and out of the Patient/Carer's world, but forget about the promises of support as soon as they return to their own lives.

Ostriches   Relatives/friends who simply cannot deal with the illness.

Stick their heads in the sand, get on with their life, and offer very little support.

Desperate for everything back to normal asap, firmly believing that they will simply pick up where they left off with Patient once recovered.

Bullets   As soon as news spreads re Severe ME, Patient/Carer will not see these guys for dust.

Good time friends who will not stick around during the bad times.

The Ugly:

Doubting   Pretty self-explanatory, these guys prefer to think that the Patient

Thomas's   is making it all up; why? Because then they have a way out, and don't have to feel guilty about not helping or supporting.

Shallow individuals who prefer to ignore the evidence of the experts and convince themselves that they know better.

Brick Walls Dangerous group of people.

Make all the right noises but never really take in what Carer/Patient tells them about the illness, particularly the need for pacing, caution and never pushing Patient to their limit.

In the recovery phase, they will push the Patient too far too fast, not heeding any of the Carer's advice, ignoring the Patient's limitations and are often responsible for major relapses.

Energy Stressful people who literally sap the energy out of the Patient.

Vampires Needy, self-centred individuals who probably leaned on the Patient pre-ME and intend to continue to do so, despite their illness.

'Takers', not 'Givers' and pose real threat to Patient's recovery.

WASPs They have never had Severe ME. They have never cared for a Severe ME Patient 24/7 month after month, year after year. They have never had any specialist ME training. And yet, in their own minds, they believe they know everything.

They prefer to offer up erroneous advice, and be aggressive and confrontational when it is ignored or challenged; in short, they are a source of HUGE stress, at a time when everyone else is trying to reduce stressors on the Patient/Carers and be supportive and helpful. Very dangerous to Patient's chances of improving.

Chapter 9: What do you say to someone with Severe ME? What can you do to help them?

So, now that you have decided what kind of supporter you want to be, let's look first at what you don't say, what you don't do for someone with Severe ME:

- **Don't be awkward and distant**. It's unfair to make the Patient feel uncomfortable just because you are. If you don't know what to say to them, just say so, be honest.

- **Don't say 'Get Well Soon'**. Of course, that is what everyone wants to happen, none more so than the Patient; but be realistic, if you want to say anything along these lines, just say something like 'you **will** get better, in your own time, when your body is ready, just take it one day at a time, you **will** get better'.

- **Don't make hurtful, ignorant statements like**:

'Pull yourself together; you have to push yourself more'

'You're simply not trying hard enough to get well'

'This time ill will be character building for you, it will make you stronger as a person'

'Well you should find something better to do with your life than lying in bed, staring out of the window at the sky'
(yes, really, a relative said this to me when I was physically incapable of doing anything else.)

'This is God's will'

'I know just how you feel' (unless you have had Severe ME.)

'You look well'

'Are you sure you're not just burnt out?'

'Come on, you can do more than that'
(if the Patient has told you they can chat for 1 minute, then that is how long you stay, don't push them beyond their limit)

'Tired eh? Blimey, you should have a go at my job and looking after three kids, now that's what I call fatigue.'

- **Don't avoid them if they are capable of having short visits**. Their illness is not contagious and if people do stay away, the Patients feel so isolated, so alone, like everyone has given up on them.

- **Likewise, if they are just too ill to receive visitors, then do not take it personally**. Of course, the Patient longs to see their friends and relatives, but if a 5-minute visit from you makes them even more exhausted and even more in pain, then don't hassle the Carer who has told you the Patient is just not up to visits yet. This is not about what you need, this is what is best for the Patient, and if you love them, then listen and learn from what the Carer is telling you.

- When you write to them (or visit them), **don't pretend like nothing has changed**. It has; they are ill, and you pretending that they everything is normal is not helpful.

- **Be sensitive**. If your life is going really well, **don't twitter on about how great everything is for you,** how you are the happiest you have ever been, how fantastic your life is etc; ok, the Patient knows that life goes on outside their bedroom's walls and is pleased that life is good for you, but don't rub their nose in your good fortune, be sensitive.

- Likewise, **don't twitter on about all your problems**, don't add to your loved one's worries, they really do have enough on their plate at the moment.

- **Don't make promises then break them** eg if you promise to write to them every week, don't just do it for a few weeks, get bored and then stop, this really is very hurtful.

- **Don't stop writing to the Patient just because you hear that he/she is too ill to read** and having to lay in a blacked-out room; the Carer can still tell them about your card/letter. When I was unable to read, my husband would always tell me when someone had sent me a card/note/email message and I would always ask him to place the card/letter/message under my pillow – it felt nice to be close to the friend/relative who had taken the trouble to keep writing to me, it gave me a lot of strength.

- **Don't drone on about what worked for your friend's moderately affected second-cousin-twice-removed, or for the person you read about in the newspaper,** who was ill for a few months with extremely Mild ME, tried a bit of Graded Exercise and Cognitive Behavioural Therapy and bobs your uncle, fully recovered – it is **NOT** helpful. Each ME Patient is unique and the recovery process for Severe ME is totally different from that of Mild/Moderate ME.

If you are struggling to get your head around this, just think about **Diabetes**, a medical condition in which the amount of glucose (sugar) in the blood is too high because the body cannot use it properly.

There are two main types of Diabetes:

- Type I Diabetes
- Type 2 Diabetes

Type I Diabetes develops if the body is unable to produce any insulin, and Diabetics therefore have to have injections of insulin every single day. If you have Type 1 Diabetes, your insulin injections are vital to keep you alive and you must have them every day.

Type 2 Diabetes develops when the body can still make some insulin, but not enough, or when the insulin that is produced does not work properly. Type 2 Diabetes is often treated first and foremost with lifestyle changes such as a healthier diet, weight loss and increased physical activity, the main aim being to achieve blood glucose levels as near normal as possible.

- One illness, two types, two very different treatments. Just like Severe ME and Mild/Moderate ME. Get the picture?

- And do remember to support your loved one just as you would a person with Diabetes. A person with Type 1 Diabetes is wholly unable to produce the insulin that he/she needs to regulate their blood sugar levels; in much the same way, a Patient with Severe ME is wholly unable to produce the energy he/she needs to function normally.

- You would never dream of encouraging a Type 1 Diabetic to skip their daily insulin injection, eat a dozen sugary doughnuts, or not eat anything for hours, of course not, because you have a level of understanding and appreciate what Type 1 Diabetics have to do to stay well and so you support them 100%.

- So, remember to do the same with your loved one who has Severe ME………. whatever they have to do to improve, give them your support and understanding, 100% of the time.

- **Don't think about the Patient constantly but never let them know – they are not telepathic**. If you don't know what to say/ write, just get a little card and write three simple words 'Thinking of You'.

- When the Patient moves from the chronic to the recovery stage of the illness, and starts to make baby steps of progress, **do not pressurise them into doing something that you want them to do before they are strong enough**, eg attend family event/ wedding/christening/birthday party.

- A highly emotional, physically and mentally draining event is a sure-fire way to a relapse – do really want that on your conscience?

- And when they do start to make progress, congratulate them on every single, tiny step they take, literally.

- Encouragement and support made such a big difference to my recovery; when one manages to stand for 5 seconds, or lift one spoonful of food, or writes one character of the alphabet, or walks 5 paces, it is very easy to feel downhearted and totally daunted at just how much one has to rebuild.

- For me, it felt like I'd found myself standing at the bottom of Everest, looking up towards the summit and wondering how the hell I was going to get up there; and even when I had started to make real progress and was able to sit for eg 10 minutes unsupported, walk for 50 paces, stand for 1 minute; even then, I had to dig deep within myself to will myself on, and on days when it just seemed too hard, too hopeless, that's when my family and friends' support and unerring encouragement drove me on. Their total faith in me and that I could and would improve, well, that gave me the strength to go on, making the ascent of my own personal Everest.

- **So, when you write to them, or visit them, do make a big deal about their progress, because it is a big deal,** eg you could write/say something like:

"I heard that you can write your signature now – that is SO brilliant, I know just how hard that must have been to rebuild and retrain the muscles in your arm and hand to do that - well done you."

Or

"I heard that you can feed yourself now lying down – well done you, really proud of ya. It must feel good to be reclaiming your independence – I know you've got a long way to go yet, but just remember that you have started, you are going in the right direction now, and I will be with you every step of the way, supporting you and willing you on".

Or

"We heard that you can now listen to 1 minute of TV now with your eyes closed – wow, what an achievement. We know how hard it must be to re-train your brain to do that, and we know how much you must long to just be able to sit and watch your fave programme on TV like everyone else; but that time will come, just keep doing what you are doing and know that we are SO proud of you, of your strength, your determination and your willpower. Hang in there kiddo, and know that we are thinking of you"

Or

"Wow, I heard that you had your first shower in 2 years at the weekend. My god, that must have felt good."

- **When they are strong enough to see you, do not talk at a million miles per hour** – their brain function will take time to improve, so talking at a relaxed rate will be much easier for them. Likewise, do not crash down on their bed and give them a huge hug - their muscles/joints are very painful and jolts will really hurt them. If in doubt, ask. Just ask them if you can give them a kiss/hug or is it ok for you to just hold their hand gently while you visit.

- **Don't be upset if the Patient asks you to leave during a visit,** they have probably spotted a couple of warning signals from their body/brain and need to rest – it's nothing personal, it's just that their precious energy stores may run down very, very quickly.

Likewise, if their Carer comes in and asks you to leave, don't get annoyed with them either, they live this illness alongside the Patient 24/7, they can spot warning signs a thousand miles off, they know when the Patient needs to rest. **If you are asked to leave, LEAVE.**

Ok, now let's look at some examples of what you do say to the Patient, what you can do for them?

- First of all, tell them that they have done absolutely nothing to deserve this terrible illness;

- There is still so little advice, so few medical specialists out there for this group of sufferers, that Severely affected ME Patients end up mentally beating themselves up, convincing themselves that they must have done something to cause this illness, because no one tells them any different. **Make sure that they know that they have done absolutely nothing wrong. Severe ME is not their fault.**

- Tell them (verbally or written word) that you are there for them, by their side as they fight this illness, that **you are in it for the long haul,** and you will be there at that final finishing line, waiting with a bottle of bubbly to celebrate.

- **Do put yourselves in their shoes, think long and hard about what life must be like for your loved one**; think about all the harsh realities of Severe ME; I know it is terribly upsetting to think about what they are having to endure, but you really do need to if you want to offer them and their Carer strength, understanding and compassion through this terrible illness.

- **Even if they are unable to talk they might like company in their bedroom**. If they are not light sensitive, maybe you could just sit in a chair, hold their hand, and just read quietly or listen to your iPod.

- **Do drop them a line, regularly, even if they cannot read it themselves, the Carer can read it out to them.** I was fortunate to have many friends and relatives that wrote to me regularly, and one dear pal wrote to me every week for the entire duration of my illness; even when she knew that I could not read them, still they came, her constancy giving me immense strength to fight on.

But even if you not organised person, go out and buy say, 12 nice cards, one per month for the coming year, stamp and address the envelope, write on top left of envelope January, February, march etc, and write inside something suitable, like

'Just to let you know that I am thinking of you' Lots love xxx

Or

'Hang in there, kiddo, you will come through this, I know you will' Lots love xxx

Or

'Sending you all our love and strength to help you fight this illness' Lots love xxx

You don't have to write much, you just have to let them know that your support is constant.

If you choose to write every week, or every fortnight, then do – but remember, don't start off by writing weekly for a few months, then move to fortnightly for six months, and then onto monthly after that – that just smacks of you giving up on the Patient, like they are taking too long to get better,

Decide the frequency of your cards/notes at the outset and STICK TO IT. Constancy is the key here.

- If the Patient is out of the light sensitive phase and can tolerate some light in their room, **why not make a 'Happy Thoughts' Mobile** – explain that the pictures are of all the things that the Patient will do again in the future when they have are stronger eg a dear friend of mine made one for me and hung little pictures of all the things she wanted me to think about doing again in the future, when I was better; the pictures she hung up included:

Picture of beach & shell –	to think about walking along a sandy beach
Picture of butterfly –	to think about lazy days sitting in a lovely garden
Picture of the world –	to remind me of all the places I would travel to
Picture of musical notes –	to remind me that I would dance again
Picture of sun –	to remind me that I would feel the sun on my face one day
Picture of Christmas Tree –	to remind me of fab Christmases still to come

I cannot begin to tell you how much strength that 'Happy Thoughts' Mobile gave me – lying in bed in constant pain, just being able to open my eyes for a few seconds, look up and see images of such hope… well, it got me through some very dark times.

- **Likewise, why not buy some lovely pictures for the bedroom walls** – don't have to spend a lot. That same pal cut up a Lake District Calendar, and mounted them on big pieces of paper – they were so beautiful to look at.

- **Gifts** are always nice for any Patient to receive, but it is best to **check with the Carer what would be a useful gift**

because Severe ME Patients have loads of sensitivities. Just try and think a bit outside the box. Turning up with piles of books, magazines, DVDs, and milk chocolates under your arm is not going to be much use if the Patient is light sensitive, can't read nor watch TV and is dairy intolerant is it.

Toiletries are great, but check which brands the Patient can now use; most Severe ME Patients have to be SO careful about personal care products because they become sensitive to many common ingredients. Good companies to check out include:

The Green People Company Ltd – www.greenpeople.co.uk

Pondtail Farm, Coolham Road, West Grinstead, West Sussex, RH13 8LN
Tel 01403 740350

The Healthy House Ltd – www.healthy-house.co.uk

The Old Co-op, Lower Street, Ruscombe, Stroud, Glos. GL6 6BU
Tel 0845 450 5950 or 01453 752216

Neals Yard Ltd – www.nealsyardremedies.com

Pyjamas, night wear, socks are always useful, but do check what materials/size they can wear; I found that I could not tolerate synthetic materials any more, having to opt for clothing made from pure cotton or pure wool instead. One of the loveliest gifts I received during my illness, was a large but light **pure wool blanket** from my husband – he gave it to me one Christmas telling me that if he was away from me, I should wrap myself up in my 'magic' blanket, and it would keep me safe and help me get better. To this day, I still have that blanket and if I ever suffer a setback, it is the first thing I grab to help me through.

And if your friend/relative *can* tolerate synthetic materials, soft fleecy blankets are great thoughtful presents because they are very light and easily manoeuvred by the Patient.

Flowers/plants might be nice to brighten up their bedroom, but do check with the Carer that the Patient has not developed hay fever/allergies or is sensitive to highly scented plants/flowers. When I was at my worst I could not tolerate any flowers/plants but when I moved out of my light sensitive phase into the recovery phase, some of the nicest presents people gave me were small plants or flowers for my room; stuck in bed, it was so nice to watch something grow eg hyacinth, amaryllis, crocuses and looking at some lovely flowers in a vase, marvelling at their beauty, really lifted my spirits.

Aromatherapy products might also be very helpful to some Patients. Neal's Yard (see above) has a whole range of products that might help the Patient but do check with their Carer, before spending a lot of money, that they can tolerate such products. If they can, investigate aromatherapy roll-ons, spritzers, hand creams, body lotions which contain relaxing oils that might help combat stress and improve sleep.

- One gift area that would be a great help to the Patient/Carer is the area of **specialist foods and supplements. Great place to head to is** www.sales@drmyhill.co.uk **Telephone: 01547 550 331.** Dr Myhill has great deal of experience dealing with ME Patients including those severely affected and offers a range of suitable supplements.

The Patient may well become intolerant to many things: eg sugar, wheat, gluten, lactose, tap water, and may well be having to take supplements to help his/her body heal. Listed below are the supplements that most helped me regain my health so you could easily ask the Carer if any of them might be suitable for the Patient:

Magnesium	Vitamin C (stomach friendly type)
Essential Fatty Acids	Glucosamine
Multivitamin & Minerals	Digestaid
Co Enzyme Q10	Gingko
Acetyl-L-Carnitine	Probiotics
Vitamin B12	Aloe Vera
Vitamin E	Vitamin B Complex
VegEPA	

If Patient suffering badly digestion wise, I found that capsules were best for me, which could be opened and the contents poured straight into my mouth to take with a little water.

These babies are very very expensive and asking the Carer if you could perhaps contribute/buy one of these for the Patient, well, this support would be very very welcome **(see Chapter 7, item 5, Nutritional Therapy for my preferred suppliers' details/contact details of experts who would be able to offer advice to you).** Health Shops are also a good source of information and usually stock a wide variety of specialist products, just look under Health Shops in your local Yellow Pages.

• Another gift that would really demonstrate how much you understand your loved one's illness is a gift that could help them relax:

Listed below are good sources of information and/or suppliers of CDs/tapes that could be of benefit to your loved on:

New World Music Ltd – www.newworldmusic.com
Suppliers of wide range of guided relaxation CDs, relaxing
music CDs and other relaxation related products.
New World Music, Harmony House, Hillside Road East,
Bungay, Suffolk NR35 1RX
Telephone: 01986 891 600

Angela Stevens – www.angela-stevens.co.uk
Breathe to Live CD is specifically for people with Severe
ME as the breathing exercises can be practised if bedbound.
Telephone: 01892 782 865
Email: info@angela-stevens.co.

Breathworks – www.breathworks-mindfulness.co.uk
Telephone: 0203 856 9561 or 0161 834 1110
Email: info@breathworks.co.uk
An organisation whose breathing exercises and meditations
can be done if bedbound

Audio Meditation: www.audiomeditation.co.uk

Downloadable meditations available
Telephone: 020 3286 6478
Email: info@augiomeditation.co.uk

Pain control is a complex and highly specialist area and as
such it is the Patient's GP/Consultant/Nurse who needs to
manage this area, BUT there are some gifts that might help
give your loved one some relief from the pain eg hot water
bottle, a wheatie (wheat pack heated in microwave), ice
packs, all of which I found useful – but check with Carer
first.

If the Patient is unable to talk, but can tolerate a little light
in their room, make a chart with letters of Alphabet which
Patient can use to point to in order to communicate. Or a
chart with common phrases on to help them communicate

eg Toilet, Hungry, Thirsty, Pain in arms, Pain in legs, Cold, Too hot, Scared, Need Hug, etc

Let them know (visits or written notes) that you understand how disciplined they are going to have to be in terms of energy management/pacing/grading activities to aid their recovery; and when they do start to make their first baby steps into their recovery phase, reinforce to the Patient all the things they need to do, eg

Encourage them to be a cautious tortoise NOT a hasty hare

Tell them to stick to the rules of recovery, pacing, grading, rests

Tell them to not push too hard, too fast, far better to nudge forwards steadily.

Tell them it's ok to progress in their own time, this is not a race.

Remind them to stop before symptoms flare up. Remind them that by the time they have symptoms, it's too late and a setback is looming.

Encourage them to always keep a third of their energy in reserve. Don't run their
Batteries down to zero.

Tell them to be disciplined.

Encourage them to stick to their BASELINES (the activities they can achieve regularly <u>without</u> exacerbating their symptoms)

Remember that one of the most bewildering aspects of Severe ME is the 'delayed reaction' aspect so reinforce that

message to your loved one; remind them that if they push themselves too far, if the overdo things and exceed their baselines, they will pay for it later.

When you are with them, ask them what their baselines are eg,

How long can we chat for today?
How long can you sit for today?
How many paces can you walk today?
How long can you stand for today?
How long can I push you in your wheelchair today?

Ask them their baselines, and then keep an eye on the time and get up and say your goodbyes as soon as that baseline has been met.

When I started to improve, I cannot tell you how much it helped to surround myself with those friends and relatives who had really made an effort to try and understand the whole illness. Recovering from Severe ME is such a lengthy and frustratingly slow process for the Patient, and constantly having to check your watch, monitor your energy levels can become so very intrusive, that sometimes the Patient just wants to scream and rage against the huge discipline that is needed to recover.

This is where your support can really make a difference – when you are with your loved one, why don't you take responsibility for watching the clock, you take responsibility for asking them if they need a rest, you take responsibility for telling other visitors to talk more slowly/more quietly if you think it's all getting too boisterous.

- And in the same vein, ask the Carer to explain to you what warning signs you should be watching out for in the Patient. To give you an idea here is a list of <u>my</u> early external warning signals:

Face drains of colour
Head/shoulders drop
Eyes become fixed/dazed
Clumsy or uncoordinated
Limbs jerk/twitch
Legs buckle/collapse
Unable to move limbs
Dark, dark circles under eyes
Unable to tolerate bright light/
Unable to tolerate noise
Slurred speech
Words come out all jumbled up
Use wrong word or work in wrong context
Get confused
Unable to follow conversation
Unable to speak
Unable to stand up
Unable to feed self

Just check with Carer is any of these apply to your loved one; if not, ask what their warning signs are and watch out for them. If, for example, you are talking to the Patient and their words come out jumbled up and don't make much sense, ask the Patient if their brain is getting tired and suggest that maybe they need a rest. Even if they don't need a full 30-minute rest, suggest that they just have a quiet 5 minutes and do some deep breathing exercises whilst you wander off for a while.

- Never forget that one of the most bewildering aspects of Severe ME is that of ***delayed reaction.***

Once they are strong enough you might find yourself visiting the Patient and they look absolutely fine, chatting away, laughing, joking with you, chatting to you, way over the time allowed and when you leave you think to yourself *"well, that was really lovely, so good to see him/her so well "*; but if the Patient talks to you too much and exceeds his/her visit baselines, what you **won't** see afterwards are the days/weeks that he/she has to lay curled up in bed, limbs like lead, migraine, foggy brain, feeling like a breathing corpse once more,

Delayed reaction - remember, this is a hellish part of Severe ME, and your loved one will be vulnerable to this reaction throughout their illness and so really try to help them by **always** checking with them what their baseline is for eg chatting, walking, sitting, standing etc, and then encourage them to stick to their baselines and avoid setbacks/relapses stuck in bed again.

A great phrase one of my friends used to say to me to encourage me to be disciplined was **'remember, Cathy, if you overdo it now, you WILL pay for it later, it's just is not worth it'.** Great friend, great advice, advice that could so easily help your loved one be disciplined too.

Chapter 10: What do you say to the Carers? What can you do to help them?

When someone becomes ill with Severe ME, their recovery becomes the sole focus for family and friends, and quite rightly so: what can I do… how can I help… what should I say…what should I do…what can I get…how can I support them…your list of questions is endless.

But it is vital to the Patient's chances of improvement' that family and friends remember to offer unconditional support to the Patient's <u>Carer</u>(s) too, both practically and emotionally, because without their Carer's constant care, love and help around the clock, the Patient has absolutely no chance of ever regaining their health.

The relationship of the main Carer(s) to the Patient can take many forms – they may be the Patient's parent, son/daughter, husband/wife, partner, sister/brother, grandparent, friend, relative; there may be one Carer only or one main Carer and one/two in support; they may be young or old, they may have to work, they may not; they may have medical training, they may not; they may have experience of caring for an ill person, they may not; but one thing that all Carers of Severe ME Patients have in common is their absolute devotion to the Patient and to doing all they can to ease their pain and suffering, to fight to get the medical help they need, and be there with them every hellish step of the way. Carer(s) put their own life on hold, they push their own needs to one side, they carry the burden without complaint and they pay little attention to their own health – so this is where you, their family and friends **MUST** step in and help them carry this heavy load.

Obviously, there will be a large crossover of advice from the previous Patient-based advice section, so let's recap on the main areas of advice that applies to helping the Carer as well as the Patient:

- **Don't be awkward and distant to the Carer**. It's unfair to make them feel uncomfortable just because you are. If you don't know what to say to them, just say so, be honest.

- **Don't patronise the Carer** and tell them that the Patient is sure to 'get well soon'. Of course, that is what everyone wants to happen, none more so than the Carer and the Patient; but be realistic, if you want to say anything along these lines, just say something like 'they **will** get better, you know, they will get better, in their own time, when their body is ready, just take it one day at a time, they **will** get better, people do you know, Catherine Saunders has'.

- **Don't make cras, hurtful, ignorant statements about the Patient like**:

'They've really got to pull themselves together; they really do have to push themselves more;

'They're obviously not trying hard enough to get well'

'This is God's will; he/she will get better when he thinks right time'

'Are you sure they're not just burnt out?'

'Come on, you know they can do more than that' (if the Carer has told you the Patient can chat for 1 minute, then that is how long you stay, don't argue with the Carer, they are the expert, not you)

'Tired eh? Blimey, they should have a go at my job and looking after three kids, now that's what I call fatigue.'

- **Be sensitive**. If your life is going really well, don't twitter on about how great everything is for you, how you are the happiest you have ever been, how fantastic your life is etc; ok, the Carer knows that everyone is getting on with their lives and is thrilled that life is good for you, but don't rub their nose in your good fortune, be sensitive that life for the Carer is pretty crap at the moment.

- **Likewise, don't twitter on about all your problems**, don't add to the Carer's worries, they really do have enough on their plate at the moment. Find someone else to moan to.

- **Don't make promises then break them** eg if you promise to do all you can to help them, don't just help out for a few weeks, get bored and then stop, this really is so very hurtful - Carers needs family and friends around them that they can totally count on, who will be there for them, for as long as it takes.

- Don't drone on about your cousin/friend's daughter/ neighbour's grandchild who has made a full recovery from Mild/Moderate ME, after a bit of graded exercise and cognitive behaviour therapy, it is **NOT** helpful. **The recovery process from Severe ME is totally different from that of Mild/Moderate ME.** Remember the difference between Diabetes I and II, two very different illnesses, two very different types of treatment; the same goes for Mild/ Moderate and Severe ME And the Carer needs to know and to hear that you understand this difference, otherwise how can they turn to you for support?

Ok, now let's move on to Carer specific advice:

Practical Support

- Looking after someone with Severe ME is exhausting, stressful and utterly draining, both physically and mentally, so one of the most helpful ways to support Carers is to **give them a break;** but remember that the kind of break that you can offer the Carer is totally dependent upon a) the stage of the Patient's illness and b) your relationship with the Patient.

- For example, when I was at my most Severe/dependent, needing to be fed by spoon, bed bathed, bedpans emptied, light sensitive and unable to talk, I truly only felt 'comfortable' with my husband, mum and mum-in-law caring for me; one loses all dignity when one is so physically disabled, and there are very very few relatives/friends that Severe ME Patients will feel able to 'let in' to see them at their worst, and indeed trust enough to believe they can care for them. So, don't take it personally if, during the most Severe phase, that your offers of help are turned down – it's just that the timings are not quite right **yet.**

- But a break does not have to mean stepping in to the main Carer's shoes 24/7 as our mums had to. At the start of my illness, when I could still talk a little and again when I started to recover and began speaking a little again, we turned to close friends and relatives who gladly made themselves available if my husband needed just a couple of hours off, or an evening, or someone to make my dinner if he had to go to a late meeting etc "Cathy-sitting" we used to call it. And most of the time, I never even saw these friends/relatives; they would just sit quietly downstairs, allowing me to feel 100% safe drifting off to sleep, knowing that if there was a problem, someone who loved me enough to give up their time was there for me if I needed them or would get me out of the house should there be a fire.

- So, make it clear to the Carer that you are very happy to do a bout of 'Patient-sitting' whenever they need you to, and if there are a few of you that feel comfortable doing this, then why don't you get a rota going, letting the Carer take a few hours off eg every Friday evening or every Saturday afternoon…you can sort out with them the timings that best suit everyone, but the important thing to remember is that once you 'sign up' for this kind of support, you can't just wriggle out of it when the fancy takes you.

- We had one 'friend' whom my husband asked to 'Cathy-sit' one Saturday evening when some old friends from New Zealand were over, so that he could just go to the pub and have a few hours off – his first Saturday night out in about 6 months – and this so-called friend rang at 5pm that evening to say that she couldn't make it, as there was a party that she wanted to go to. So, remember, if you commit to helping out in this way, commit 100%, or don't commit at all.

- Now let's move on to another area in which Carers would really appreciate some help – running the household. If you live locally, perhaps you can help out with some of the **household chores** and take some of the weight off the Carer's shoulders, eg

  - weekly shopping
  - laundry
  - ironing
  - mowing the lawn/tending the garden
  - cooking (even if the Patient's food is too complicated for you to make because of all their food sensitivities/allergies, you could always cook eg a casserole for the Carer to pop in the freezer)
  - cleaning

- If there are a few of you that live locally, perhaps you could organise a **rota system** for some of the above; why not get all of you together and decide who is going to do what and when; and remember whatever each of you 'signs up' to do, you are in this for the long haul, so if four of you decide to take it in turns to pick up a bag of laundry every Thursday evening, to wash and iron and deliver back to the Carer on Tuesday evening, then you may be doing this for quite some time.

- If the Patient/Carer is a parent, **helping out with their kids** would be a huge help eg taking/picking them up from school, ferrying them around to their various clubs/activities, cooking their tea for them, having them stay for a sleepover or cooking up a load of kids' meals for the freezer.

- Likewise, if the Patient/Carer was involved with looking after an elderly relative nearby, maybe you could take that burden off their shoulders and step in to **helping out with their eg elderly mother/grandmother.** Really have a think about what the Patient/Carer's responsibilities were before Severe ME, and ask yourself if you could take on any of those responsibilities until they can resume a normal life.

- If you do not live nearby but are very, very close to the Patient/Carer and desperate to help out in a practical way, would you be prepared to get together with some of your other relatives/friends in the same position and eg stump up some cash to pay for a eg **weekly cleaner/gardener/ ironer for the household**? Money is usually very tight in most households hit by Severe ME, as often a salary has been lost (Patient's and/or Carer's) and the costs involved in caring for the Patient can escalate rapidly, eg special foods/ supplements/complementary therapies etc.

- Alternatively, if you live far away, could you commit some of your free time and eg **visit one weekend every three months**? If you could, then you could be really useful, eg giving the Carer a break/giving the house a spring clean/ tidying the garden/doing a big food shop/washing and ironing. And be prepared to offer to stay at a B&B/Hotel – the Patient may just not be able to cope with the extra noise in the house with you staying.

- Another very useful way to help the Patient and the Carer(s) is the area of **Researching Severe ME and treatments**. There are still so few medical professionals that truly understand Severe ME, that finding out what to do for the best for the Patient is both time consuming and emotionally draining…and frankly, the Carer has their hands full just trying to get the Patient through each day. So, if you feel at home on the internet, maybe this is an area where you can offer your services.

See Section 7 for contact details of the main sources of information which I found very useful and Page 104 for a list of Books that proved very useful.

• So get on to the websites, join the associations, look at the latest research, buy a book from my list on page 65 etc, and try and summarise your findings for the Carer; but remember, each Severe ME Patient is unique, so what works for one Patient may or may not work for your loved one; **remember that finding out what your loved one needs to improve is rather like trying to complete a complex jigsaw puzzle or sometimes it can feel as if you are trying to find your way through a maze…….so be Patient**, if you suggest something to the Carer which does not work, don't take it personally, just get straight back into the sources of information, do some more research, and keep going until you find something that does help them. Work with the Carer, take on board their feedback – they are the ones who understand the uniqueness of your loved one's illness – and just keep searching, you <u>will</u> find things that will help them.

• **Keeping everyone up to date with the Patient's condition is another area which you could really help the Carer with.**

Imagine how time consuming it is for the Carer to have to keep updating all the relatives and friends re Patient's status/progress…the phone ringing constantly… repeating the update to all the well-meaning callers at the end of another exhausting day. And then, when the Carer finds he/she simply does not have the energy left to call people back, imagine the guilt they then feel, on top of everything else they are carrying.

So why not step in and take over this responsibility. If you are internet savvy, get the email addresses off the Carer, and do a short weekly email to relatives/friends to let them know how the Patient is doing. If you prefer to talk to people direct, why not involve a few other relatives/friends and each take responsibility to ring say 6 people and update them every week. It really would be a huge weight off the Carer's mind, knowing that everyone knows what is going on.

Emotional Support

- **Carers of Severe ME Patients go through hell but they often keep the harsh realities of what they have to cope with on a daily basis, locked away deep inside, telling everyone that *"they are fine"*, when asked how they are doing.**

- Having read this Book, ask yourself how on earth could anyone caring for a Severe ME Patient be 'fine', watching their eg son/daughter or husband/wife in pain, bed-bound, suffering so much just to get through each day, unable to talk, to walk or see daylight, with little or no medical help... **so even though it is easier for you to take their answer at face value, remember, Carers are anything but fine. They are an emotional mess.**

- Take my husband, for example, when I became so Severely ill, it must have felt like I had died; the fun loving, energetic, vibrant woman he fell in love with had disappeared completely, leaving behind nothing but a breathing corpse, a helpless soul whom he had to nurse like a baby, dependent upon him for everything, absolutely everything. True, I was not dead, but then neither was I truly alive, just a shell of the woman he once shared his life with.

How could he possibly be fine?

So how can you support Carers emotionally?

- Well, this is going to depend a lot on the personality of the Carer and your relationship with them. If you are very close to them, and they are an open kind of character, **make sure you tell them often that they can lean on your shoulder any time, that you are happy to listen to them offload and that anything they confide in you goes no further.**

- If, however, they are the kind of person who does not open up readily, then respect that and just say something along the lines of *'look, I know that you aren't fine, how could you be. Just know that if you ever want to talk/cry/scream/rant then I am here for you'*. And don't just say it once; say it regularly so that the Carer knows that your offer of support is real, not merely empty words.

- And however, upset the whole situation makes you feel, however much you miss the Patient and are devastated by what has happened to them, **do NOT turn to the Carer for comfort** – find someone else to lean on, Carers don't have anything left to give.

- And if you are really worried about the stress and strain that the Carer is under, remember that there is support out there, whether it is financial, emotional or practical – the key is knowing how to access it. Carers UK and The Princess Royal Trust for Carers operate advice lines, run local support groups, and provide information re services and benefits. Also, the Patient's Local Authority may have local Carers Groups and you could definitely investigate this for the Carer. And don't forget to find out if there is a local ME Group in their area – this would be a great support, to be amongst people who truly understand what they are going through (contact Action for ME or The ME Association as a start point to find out what services are available in the Carer's area).

Carers UK – www.carersuk.org

Carers UK 020 7378 4999
Carers Wales 029 2081 1370
Carers Scotland 0141 445 3070
Carers Northern Ireland 02890 439 843

- Investigate whether there is a local **Disabled Living Centre** near them – they can give the Carer advice on equipment which might ease the physical burden of caring. Visit www. disabledliving.co.uk and have a look at the Equipment (Equipz) section. Also see if there is a Mobility shop in their area, they can be a great source of help and information.

- I have already touched upon how a short break can make a huge difference to the Carer. As well as friends and relatives rallying around to provide back up, it is worth contacting Carers UK to see if there is any help available for a few hours care a week.

- Lastly, remember that the Carer would also welcome thoughtful acts of kindness from you, just as much as the Patient – eg

  - a little card to let them know you are thinking of them too
  - a bunch of flowers
  - a box of chocolates
  - a 'Calm' aromatherapy Spritzer or some relaxing bubble bath from Neal's Yard (www.nealsyardrememedies. com)
  - a bottle of good Multivitamin & Mineral tablets and/or B Complex to help with stress (www.biocare.co.uk)
  - a bottle of wine

- a nice home cooked casserole
- a relaxation CD
- www.newworldmusic.com

- Another way you might be able to help Carers is by **taking their minds of things, distracting them for a short while**. Let's just say for example that someone is 'babysitting' the Patient for a few hours and the Carer is meeting up with you and a few others at eg pub/restaurant.

Now, obviously, you are all going to ask how the Patient is, that's fine, absolutely natural and yes, of course, maybe some people there will have some more questions about the illness/recovery/treatments etc, but if this line of conversation is going on for more than say half an hour, then just lean in to the Carer, subtly, and ask them if they want to carry on talking about ME or would they prefer to have their minds taken off the situation for a few hours and talk about something else.

Sometimes the Carer may need to escape the nightmare of Severe ME for a few hours to find the strength to return to it.

<u>Chapter 11 – Conclusion</u>

So, at long last, here I am writing the final page of this Book

I truly hope that I have succeeded in explaining the harsh reality of Severe ME and addressed some of the many questions, worries and fears you have about what is happening to your friend/relative.

All that is left to me now is to ask you to share this knowledge with anyone who is ignorant of these facts so that the thousands of Severe ME Patients out there who feel invisible, and abandoned, along with their Carers, begin to receive all the help, understanding, support and compassion they deserve.

About the Author

Catherine Saunders had a successful career in Marketing working with blue-chip Clients such as Pepsi-Cola, Colgate-Palmolive, Heinz, Royal Mail, Cussons, Sony and Guinness, until she became ill with Very Severe ME

She lives with her husband in Cheshire and still manages her condition carefully including the dreaded setbacks which are part and parcel of a fluctuating illness like ME; Catherine and her husband take life one day at a time, thankful to have each other and the wonderful friends and family who support them and hope that one day, soon, a cure will be found to finally help the 15-30 million Millions Missing ME patients around the world.

Bibliography & Recommended Reading

Myhill, Dr Sarah, *Diagnosis and Treatment of Chronic Fatigue Syndrome*
Puri, Professor Basant K., *Chronic Fatigue Syndrome*, Hammersmith Press 2005
Cox, Diane L, *Occupational Therapy and Chronic Fatigue Syndrome* 2000
Agombar, Fiona, *Beat Fatigue with Yoga*, Thorsons, 2002
Ali, Dr Mosaraf, *The Integrated Health Bible*, Vermillion 2001
Macintyre, Dr Anne, *ME Post Viral Fatigue Syndrome How to Live with It,* Thorsons 1988
Vries, Jan De, Viruses, *Allergies and The Immune System*, Mainstream Publishing 1995
Valerie Ann Worwood, *The Fragrant Pharmacy, A Complete Guide to Aromatherapy & Essential Oils*
Kenny, Timothy, *Living with Chronic Fatigue Syndrome*, Thunder's Mouth Press 1994

Perrin, Dr Raymond, *The Perrin Technique*, Hammersmith Press 2008

Hurrell, Janet, *The Journey through ME,* AuthorHouse 2006

McTaggart, Lynne, The Candida and ME Handbook, Copyright 2001. What Doctors Don't Tell You Limited

Worwood, Valerie Ann, *The Fragrant Pharmacy*, Bantam Books 1991

Courteney, Hazel, *500 of the most important ways to stay younger longer*, Cico Books 2003

Glenville, Dr Marilyn, *The Nutritional Health Handbook for Women*, Piatkus 2001

McKenna, Dr John, *Alternative to Antibiotics*, Gill & Macmillan 1996

Mervyn, Leonard, *Thorsons Complete Guide to Vitamins and Minerals*, Thorsons 1989

Clyton, Dr Paul, *Health Defence*, Accelerated Learning Systems 2001

Straten, Michael van, *Super Boosters*, Mitchell Beazley 2000

Selby, Anna, *Miracle Foods*, Hamlyn 2001

Vicki Edgson & Ian Marber, *The Food Doctor*, Collins & Brown 1999

Simpson, Liz, *The Book of Crystal Healing*, Gaia Books 1997

Joe Griffin & Ivan Tyrrell, *Human Givens*, HG Publishing 2004

Nikolic, Seka, *You Can Heal Yourself*, Sidgwick & Jackson 2006

Vries, Jan De, *Neck and Back Problems*, Mainstream Publishing 2004

Philips, Alasdair & Jean, *Killing Fields in the Home,* Green Audit Books 1999

Hay, Louise L, *The Power is Within You*, Eden Grove Editions 1991

Gottlyb, Bill, *Alternative Cures*, Rodale 2000

Appendix I

The ME Association – www.meassociation.org.uk

A leading ME Charity, The ME Association has compiled a list of **NHS Specialist Services round the UK** available to ME patients on their website: http://www.meassociation.org.uk/nhsspecialistservices/ To help spread the details of sources of help, the list is set out below. When contacting, a sensible question to ask is whether their team have any experience of treating Very Severe ME Patients (Grade 4-5) or whether their experience is only of treating Mild to Moderate ME Patients (Grades 1-3).
(List correct as at October 2017 and with great thanks to The ME Association)

Part 1:
NHS Clinical Network Coordinating Centres (CNCCs)
There now appear to be eight Clinical Network Coordinating Centres (CNCCs) across England – championing the development of services and improved clinical care in their area. Each CNCC has an individual, named clinical champion or network co-ordinator. Advice to patients, GPs and carers about services is available from the Network Co-ordinator at each centre.
Northern Region
(North of Tyne, South of Tyne, Teesside, Durham and Darlington, Cumbria North).
Clinical champion: Dr Gavin Spickett, consultant clinical immunologist, The Newcastle upon Tyne Hospital NHS Trust, Royal Victoria Infirmary, Queen Victoria Road, Newcastle upon Tyne NE1 4LP.

North, East and West Yorkshire
Clinical champion: Dr Hiroko Akagi, Consultant Liaison Psychiatrist, Leeds and West Yorkshire CFS/ME Service, Therapy Suite, First Floor, Newsam Centre, Seacroft Hospital, York Road, Leeds LS14

6WB, Tele: 0113 85 56330 / 0113 85 56331 / 0113 85 56334 or email: cfsme.lypft@nhs.net.

South Yorkshire and North Derbyshire
Michael Carlisle Centre, Lyndhurst Road, Sheffield S11 9BJ Service manager and lead occupational therapist: Anne Nichol. Tel: 0114 226 3232 Fax: 0114 354 0124 Email: sheffieldcfsmeservice@nhs.net This is a specialist therapy service for people affected by ME/CFS across South Yorkshire and North Derbyshire. The catchment area covers Sheffield, Rotherham, Doncaster, Barnsley, North Derbyshire County and Hardwick Clinical Commissioning Groups. Referral guidance and summary information can be found by searching for CFS and/or ME at www.sheffieldccgportal.co.uk

East Midlands
Network co-ordinator: Rehabilitation, Level 1, Royal Derby Hospital, Uttoxeter Road, Derby DE22 3NE. Tel: 01332 786657

North London/Essex/Sussex and Hertfordshire
Joint clinical champions: Professor Peter D White, Professor of Psychological Medicine at Barts and the London School of Medicine and Dentistry, and Dr Maurice Murphy, consultant in immunology and HIV medicine.
The Chronic Fatigue Syndrome Service, St Leonard's Hospital, Block A, Ground Floor, Nuttal Street, London N1 5LZ. Tel: 0203 738 7230, email: **chronic.fatique@nhs.net** (sic) (for people living in North London, Essex, Sussex and Hertfordshire).

South West London/Surrey (Sutton)
Clinical champion: Dr Amolak Bansal, Department of Immunology, St Helier Hospital, Wrythe Lane, Carshalton, Surrey SM5 1AA. Tel: 0208 296 4152
Dorset/Hampshire and Isle of Wight
Clinical champion: Dr Selwyn Richards, consultant rheumatologist, Poole Hospital NHS Trust, Longfleet Road, Poole, Dorset BH15 2JB). Tel: 01929 557560

Avon, Wiltshire, Gloucestershire, Somerset
Clinical Champion: Dr Hazel O'Dowd, Bristol CFS/ME Service, The Lodge, Cossham Hospital, Lodge Road, Bristol BS15 1LF. Telephone: 0117 3408390, Fax: 0117 3408466 Email: CFS. NHS.Bristol@nbt.nhs.uk

---

Part 2:
Adult NHS ME/CFS Specialist Services in England

Greater London

South London and Maudsley NHS Trust
Chronic Fatigue Research and Treatment Unit, Mapother House, De CrespignyPark,LondonSE58AZ.Tel:02032285075.Fax:02032285074 Our multidisciplinary team includes psychiatrists, psychologists, physiotherapists, psychotherapists, doctors and researchers. Director: Professor Trudie Chalder. We offer evidence-based treatment that is routinely evaluated. Our aim is to increase the person's functioning and reduce the severity and impact of their symptoms. We also offer assessment and treatment for people with fatigue associated with chronic diseases like rheumatoid arthritis, multiple sclerosis, HIV or cancer. We offer diagnostic specialist assessment, routine blood tests, CBT and Graded Exercise Therapy Eligibility: 10+ years (we work in conjunction with our child and adolescent service), long lasting fatigue, profound disability, disturbed sleep pattern. We accept referrals from consultant psychiatrists, community mental health teams, CAMHS, GPs and GP consortia from all over the UK apart from those areas which have their own local adult services.

South West London/Surrey (Sutton)
Sutton/St Helier Chronic Fatigue Service, The Malvern Centre, St Helier Hospital, Wrythe Lane, Carshalton, Surrey SM5 1AA. Tel: 0208 296 4152
The team comprises: Dr Amolak Bansal, consultant immunologist; Karen Tweed, clinical nurse specialist; Dr Zoe Clyde, consultant clinical psychologist; Dr Yasmin Mullick, Clinical Psychologist; Clare Inglis, physiotherapist.

Royal Free Hospital
The Fatigue Service, Department of Infection and Immunity, Royal Free Hospital, Pond Street, London NW3 2QG. Tel: 0203 758 2000 (switchboard)
Consultant: Dr Gabrielle Murphy (part-time).
Areas covered: Barnet, Camden, Enfield, Haringey and Islington.

Royal London Hospital for Integrated Medicine
Adult Chronic Fatigue Service, Royal London Hospital for Integrated Medicine (formerly the Royal London Homeopathic Hospital), 60 Great Ormond Street, London WC1N 3HR. Patient inquiries – tel: 0203 448 2000. GP inquiries: tel: 0203 448 2000, fax: 0203 448 2004, email: rlhimpatients@uclh.nhs.uk (not for referrals). Service Manager: Loretta Chinwokwu Consultants: Dr Saul Berkovitz, Dr Helmut Roniger and Dr

Christian Hasford.
This is the adult service for University College Hospital, London as a whole. Although physically based within the RLHIM, it is not a homeopathic service but offers all interventions recommended by the National Institute for Health and Clinical Excellence in their ME/CFS Guideline – including consultant physician assessment, activity management, exercise and psychological interventions including medical hypnosis, autogenic training and CBT. Clinical lead: Dr Saul Berkovitz. The team consists of three consultant physicians, a senior nurse practitioner, occupational therapist, physiotherapist and dietitian. The team also can advise on appropriate complementary medicine interventions and, in some cases, provide them – such as acupuncture for chronic widespread muscle pain. Referrals through the patient's GP or NHS hospital consultant]

St Bartholomew's Hospital
The Chronic Fatigue Syndrome Service, St Leonard's Hospital, Block A, Ground Floor, Nuttal Street, London N1 5LZ (see information under 'Clinical Network Coordinating Centres'). Tel: 0203 738 7230, email: chronic.fatique@nhs.net (sic) (for people living in North London, Essex, Sussex and Hertfordshire).

Hillingdon Hospital, Uxbridge

Greenacres Centre, Hillingdon Hospital, Pield Heath Road, Middlesex UB8 3NB, tel: 01895 279 374, fax: 01895 279 046, emaiL: hillingdoncfsme@cnwl@nhs.net
Service administrator: Renuka Mahabeer.
We accept referrals from GPs and other NHS professionals on behalf of patients within the boroughs of Harrow, Hillingdon, Hammersmith & Fulham, Kensington, Chelsea & Westminster, Brent, Ealing and Hounslow.All referrals must be accompanied by a complete set of blood results as detailed on our referral form.

Bath and Wiltshire

Bath Centre for Fatigue Services (formerly known as Adult Fatigue Management or Bath and Wiltshire CFS/ME Service), Royal National Hospital for Rheumatic Diseases, Upper Borough Walls, Bath, Somerset BA1 1RL.Tel: 01225 473456 Fax 01225 473411 Email: admin.bcfs@rnhrd.nhs.uk
Our ME/CFS service provides a local, regional and national service for adults with ME/CFS and acts in a specialist advisory capacity for professionals working with adults with the condition. We are a specialist team committed to delivering evidence-based quality services for people with fatigue. All treatment plans are agreed jointly with our patients based on their individual needs. We work closely with service users to review, develop and deliver our services. We currently have eight service users as expert educators who input to our group treatment programmes. Our service provides specialist assessment clinics and treatment based on the National Institute for Health and Clinical Excellence (NICE) guidelines for the management of ME/CFS. We provide group programmes or individual sessions if required.

Bedfordshire

Bedfordshire Chronic Fatigue Service, Disability Research Centre, Poynters House, Poynters Road, Dunstable, Bedfordshire LU5 4TP. Team co-ordinator, Jane Forbes-Pepitone; Clinical Service Manager, Dr Judith Friedman; Associate Director, Hugh Johnston.
The service can be contacted on Tuesdays (9am-1pm), Wednesdays (9am-5pm), Thursdays (9am-5pm). Tel: 01582 470 918. Fax: 01582 709 057 Email: bedscfs@sept.nhs.uk

This service is provided by the South Essex Partnership University NHS Foundation Trust and comes within the ambit of Mental Health Services. An information leaflet for service users can be downloaded

Berkshire

Berkshire Healthcare NHS Trust provide a CFS service through their Clinical Health Psychology Service.

CFS Service, Clinical Health Psychology, 25 Erleigh Road, Reading RG1 5LR. Tel: 0118 929 6474

"If you think you or someone you care about could benefit from the service please talk to your GP, hospital consultant or other healthcare professional. Unfortunately, we are not able to accept self-referrals. "Once you have been referred to us, you will be sent a letter of acknowledgement and information about any waiting times. You will be sent an initial appointment as soon as one becomes available. "Your first appointment will usually last an hour and will be an opportunity for you to discuss your current difficulties and to decide how psychology therapy could help support you." The MEA understands that home visits are being made to severely ill patients.

Bolton and Bury

The Breightmet Health Centre, Breightmet Fold Lane, Breightmet, Bolton BL2 6NT, tel: 01204 462 765, fax: 01204 462 768. Principal service lead: Simon Crozier. Manager: Michelle Wardle. The appointments are at Breightmet Health Centre if in Bolton or the Prestwich Walk-In Centre if you live in Bury. The aim of the service is to offer group and individual therapy and a domiciliary service for the housebound, in Bury and Bolton. Principal service lead: Simon Crozier. Manager: Michelle Wardle.

Birmingham and Solihull

Queen Elizabeth Hospital, The Barberry, 35 Vincent Drive, Edgbaston, Birmingham B15 2FG.

Tel: 0121 301 2280. Email: cfs-me@bsmhft.nhs.uk

The service, led by a consultant neuropsychiatrist, offers diagnosis and rehabilitation programme mostly delivered by occupational therapists and specialist nurses.

Bristol, North Somerset and Gloucestershire

Bristol CFS/ME Service, The Lodge, Cossham Hospital, Lodge Road, Bristol, BS15 1LF. Telephone: 0117 3408390. Fax: 0117 3408466. Email: CFS.NHS.Bristol@nbt.nhs.uk

"Bristol Chronic Fatigue Syndrome/ME Service is a specialist NHS Service for people with Chronic Fatigue Syndrome/ME. The clinical team includes – Occupational Therapists, Physiotherapists, Clinical Psychologists, A Counsellor."

"We offer an outpatient service to people living in Bristol, North Somerset, and Gloucestershire. We offer a combination of telephone and face-to-face contact, and a telephone counselling service is available for people who have been assessed by the Service. Part of our role is to advise and support other Health Care Professionals in the clinical management of people with CFS/ME."

"The Service can be contacted by email, telephone or by letter or fax. The best days to contact our administrator by telephone are a Monday, Wednesday or Friday."

"In 2004, North Bristol NHS Trust was selected as one of 14 specialist centres in the UK for the development of services for people diagnosed with Chronic Fatigue Syndrome/ME. The service has built up considerable expertise over the years in supporting people living with CFS/ME."

Buckinghamshire

Buckinghamshire Chronic Pain and Fatigue Management Service, Rayners Hedge, Croft Road, Aylesbury, Bucks HP21 7RD, tel: 01296 393319 (ext24). Fax: 01296392480. Email: susan.cato@buckspct.nhs.uk Clinical lead: Dr John Pimm, consultant clinical neuropsychologist. Interdisciplinary service offering cognitive behaviour therapy, graded exercise therapy and self-management outpatient programmes looking at physical, practical and psychological strategies for managing ME/CFS. The service has been running for 10 years. Referrals need to come through a medical practitioner or allied health professional e.g. GPs, hospital consultants, physiotherapists. If people live outside the area then out-of-area funding needs to be applied for.

Cambridgeshire and Peterborough

Botolph Bridge Community Health Centre, Sugar Way, Woodston, Peterborough PE2 9QB Tel: 01733 774 583 Fax: 01733 774 514 Email: cpm-tr.CFSME@nhs.net

The Cambridgeshire and Peterborough ME/CFS Team, based in Peterborough, comprises a Specialist Nurse Practitioner and three Specialist Occupational Therapists. We offer diagnosis of ME/CFS and support in management for adults aged 17+ affected by, or suspected of having ME/CFS.

We must have a referral by a GP due to a requirement for exclusionary test results. While the team is based in Peterborough, the therapists do offer follow-up appointments at two other locations in the county.

Cheshire

There are no specialist ME/CFS services in Cheshire.

Cornwall and the Isles of Scilly

Cornwall and Isles of Scilly CFS/ME Service, The Lighthouse, Royal Cornwall Hospitals Trust. Truro. TR1 3LJ. Tel: 01872 252935. Providing local clinics, home visits and group work for assessment, diagnosis, rehabilitation and reablement by a multi-disciplinary team for adults and children. The team consists of Dr Julie Thacker, Carol Wilson, Dr Lopez Chertudi, Mel Terry, Debby Reid and Cathy Jackson. Services provided are based on NICE Guideline 53. Adult referrals by GP or Consultant via paper or referral management team please.

North Cumbria

North Cumbria CFS/ME Service, Keswick Community Hospital, Crosthwaite Road, Keswick, Cumbria CA12 5HP.
Tel: 017687 245 699 Email:cfs-team@cumbria.nhs.uk
The service is led by Dr Gavin Spickett, Consultant Immunologist and CFS/ME Clinic Champion for the North of England. Therapy clinics are held in Keswick, and once a month in Carlisle.

Cumbria (South) – See entry for Lancashire and South Cumbria

Derbyshire

Tel: 01332 786657

Clinical lead: Bozena Smith, occupational therapist, Rehabilitation Centre, Royal Derby Hospital, Uttoxeter Road, Derby DE22 3NE.

Devon

South and West Devon CFS/ME Service is run on behalf of Torbay and Southern Devon Health and Care NHS Trust at the following address: 3rd Floor, Union House, Union Street, Torquay TQ1 3YA. Administrator: Louise Swann, tel: 01803 219 859 fax: 01803 219 893 email: swdevoncfsme.sdhc@nhs.net

The EXETER EAST, MID AND NORTH DEVON CFS/ME Service is based at the Arlington Centre, Whipton Hospital, Hospital Lane, Whipton, Exeter EX1 3RB, tel: 01392 208 614 The services is commissioned to provide treatment based on the NICE guidelines, Most patients will be seen by one of the two medical consultants involved to ensure that they have a correct diagnosis. Where the diagnosis is in doubt, a proper medical assessment can allow for appropriate further investigation or referral to other specialist services. At the end of the consultation, the consultant will agree a suggested plan of management which may include referral to the therapy team of the CFS/ME service together with some written suggestions to the GP about further investigations or actions to help symptoms. On occasions, it might be helpful for the consultant to see the patient at a later stage after therapy input to see if there is anything further that can be added medically in terms of help or advice.

The PLYMOUTH service is run on behalf of Sentinel Healthcare South West Community Interest Company at the following address: Express Diagnostics & Treatment Centre, Plymouth Science Park, Plymouth PL6 8BU. Administrator: Trudi, tel: 0845 155 8297
Email: PCHCIC.SentinelClinicalTreatmentService@nhs.net

The Service Manager/Senior CFS/ME Specialist for both the above services covering the whole of the South and West of Devon. The team currently consists of a medical lead Dr Robert Gardner, Senior specialist Occupational therapists, two specialist Occupational

Therapists and two administrators (as below).[SEP]The service is an adult community service providing, assessment, diagnosis and treatment for individuals suffering the complex symptoms of CFS/ME. The service is offered where appropriate to all levels of CFS/ME, mild, moderate and severe. [SEP]Along with the treatment approaches advised by NICE guidelines this service is also part of a national group auditing and implementing research and evidenced-based Mindfulness CBT approaches, to support patients psychologically with coping with this condition. The service is also able to provide extensive knowledge gained through patient experience and reporting.

Dorset

Tel: 01929 557560
This service is provided through an outpatient clinic at Wareham Community Hospital, Streche Road, Wareham, Dorset BH20 4QQ. The service – which has been supported throughout by the Dorset ME Group – celebrated its tenth anniversary in 2009. The clinical lead is Dr Selwyn Richards, a consultant rheumatologist.

Durham and Darlington

CFS/ME Service, Merrington House, Merrington Lane, Spennymoor, County Durham DL16 7UT, Tel: 01388 825700 Fax: 01388 819718 Email: cdda-tr.cfsme@nhs.net
The service only accepts referrals from GPs in Durham and Chester-le-Street, Derwentside, Dales, Darlington, and Sedgefield.

Essex
Essex-wide

Managed from Southend Hospital NHS Foundation Trust, Prittlewell Chase, Westcliff on Sea, SS0 0RY, with most of the therapy services being provided at The Tyrells Health Wing, Benfleet, Essex. Service administrator: Jenny Livemore. Tel: 01702 385 247 Fax: 01702 385 904
This service offers a consultant assessment for diagnosis, and therapy services including Graded Exercise, Pacing and Activity Management and CBT. These sessions are available

at Colchester Primary Care Centre, Broomfield Hospital in Chelmsford and in Harlow. Access to the service is via GP referral.

Essex: Queen's Hospital, Romford
Tel: 01708 435000 ext. 2647
There is a weekly NHS outpatient clinic – for new patients only – at the Queen's Hospital. Funding must be obtained by the referring GP. GPs should address referrals to Dr A Chaudhuri. Nationwide referrals are accepted.

Hampshire and the Isle of Wight
The NHS service in Southampton closed in April 2014. An NHS referral service, South Coast Fatigue (see below), is now taking referrals.
South Coast Fatigue
South Coast Fatigue, Lancaster Court, 8 Barnes Wallis Road, East Segensworth, Fareham, Hampshire PO15 5TU. Tel: 01489 668 109 Email: info@southcoastfatigue.co.uk.
Director and Specialist Occupational Therapist, Fran Hill. This is an NHS referral service offering an Interim NHS Mild to Moderate Outpatient Service to patients in West Hampshire, Fareham and Gosport, Southampton City, North Hampshire and South Eastern Hampshire. This interim service is being offered until the end of June 2015 when there will be a longer-term commissioned service in place. GPs can refer directly to South Coast Fatigue and all surgeries have a copy of the referral form. At present, once the referral has been received and screened, the pathway starts with a telephone assessment followed by a face-to-face consultation, then a mixture of telephone reviews and face-to-face appointments to go through the programme.
As part of the interim service, people can also access Mindfulness Groups, Physiotherapy and Dietician sessions.
The Isle of Wight is not part of this interim arrangement and we are advised that people need to ask their GP to apply for an Individual Funding Request (IFR).
South Coast Fatigue also has a bespoke severe service which is for people who are house/bedbound and this has to be applied for via an IFR which the GP does.

Portsmouth Chronic Fatigue Syndrome Service

Chronic Fatigue Syndrome Service, Long-Term Conditions Suite, Ground Floor, Block A, St Mary's Community Health Campus, Milton Road, Portsmouth PO3 6AD, Tel: 02392 683 386. Fax: 02392 680 201. Service lead: Rhona McGurk, clinical psychologist The Chronic Fatigue Syndrome service offers treatment programmes for people diagnosed with Chronic Fatigue Syndrome or Myalgic Encephalomyelitis (ME). This is a community-based service for adults aged 16 years and over. The team consists of a Specialist Practitioner and an Occupational Therapist. The service offers assessments to help GPs confirm diagnosis and treatment programmes aim to improve the self-management of symptoms, increase functioning and improve quality of life.

Harrogate, North Yorkshire

CFS/ME service, Briary Wing, Harrogate District Hospital, Lancaster Park Road, Harrogate HG2 7SX.
Tel 01423 553526 Fax: 01423 553586.
Julie Robinson, occupational therapist (Team Leader).
The service was set up by North Yorkshire and York Primary Care Trusts and covers Harrogate, Ripon, Skipton and surrounding areas. It hopes to expand in the future.

Hertfordshire

Hertfordshire CFS/ME and Chronic Pain Service, Maple Therapy Unit, St Albans City Hospital, Waverley Road, St Albans Hertfordshire AL3 5PN Tel: 01727 897542

Hull and East Yorkshire

A multi-disciplinary service for adult patients with a diagnosis of Chronic Fatigue Syndrome (CFS). Clarendon House, Victoria House, Park Street, Hull, HU2 8TD. Tel: 01482 617735 Fax: 01482 322211. The general contact hours for the service are 9am to 5pm, Monday-Friday. Our consultant physician is based at Hull Royal Infirmary and the therapy aspect of the service is based at the Department of Psychological Medicine. Referral to physiotherapy can be made by members of the CFS team as appropriate.

Isle of Man
Community Health Centre, Westmoreland Road, Douglas (The old Noble's Hospital site). Therapist-led service set up in 2007.

Kent and Medway
Kent and Medway CFS/ME Service, Neuropsychology Medway Admin Hub, Disablement Services Centre, Medway Maritime Hospital, Gillingham, Kent ME7 5NY. Tele: 01634 833937. "The emphasis of our service is on self-management and rehabilitation and draws on principles of cognitive behavioural therapy (CBT) and graded activity."
"Treatment is a collaborative process and the focus is always based on your needs and capabilities. The treatment programme aims to help you build on your problem-solving techniques so you can discover the most useful ways to manage and overcome your illness."

Leeds and West Yorkshire
The Leeds and West Yorkshire CFS / ME Service is based in the Therapy Suite on the first floor of the Newsam Centre and can be contacted on 0113 85 56330 / 0113 85 56331 / 0113 85 56334 or by email: cfsme.lypft@nhs.net. "Our individual treatment plans and different options for treatment help people make sense of their condition and work towards recovery."
The aims of our service are to:
– improve your quality of life – people say we are giving them their lives back
– help you on a journey towards recovery
– help you to continue in education and work if this is important to you
– help you understand your condition
– involve and support your carers, family and friends too.
Our service operates Monday to Friday, 8.30am to 4.30pm."

Leicestershire and Rutland
Referrals are currently being directed to the Brandon Unit at Leicester General Hospital, where the clinical lead is Dr Trevor Friedman, a liaison psychiatrist: Brandon Unit, Gwendolen Road, Leicester LE5 4PW, tel: 0116 225 6193 (As at December 2012, we are informed

that it was agreed that patients with M.E. were to be dealt with via neurology at the Leicester Royal Infirmary but that there are no current services available there. We suggest that patients discuss the services available with the local support group in the area – click on **this link** to find our local support group contacts page.)

Lincolnshire
CFS/ME service, Ward 14a, Grantham Hospital, 101 Manthorpe Road, Grantham, Lincolnshire, NG31 8DG. Tel: 0303 123 4000 Fax: 01476 464889 Email: lpn-tr.LincsCFS-MEService@nhs.net "The service aims to provide specialist assessment, rehabilitation interventions, and management advice from a range of disciplines. The service also aims to provide expert advice, education and support to health professionals, statutory and non-statutory organisations, service users and carers." "The CFS/ME service is a small, multidisciplinary team consisting of a consultant clinical

psychologist, a specialist occupational therapist, a senior rehabilitation assistant, a specialist physiotherapist and an assistant psychologist. Our administrative base is Grantham and District Hospital, but clinical staff are community based covering Lincolnshire."

Liverpool
The Liverpool CFS/ME Therapy Service, Ward 10, Alexandra Wing, Broadgreen Hospital L14 3LB, part of the Royal Liverpool and Broadgreen University Hospitals Trust. Tel: 0151 282 6185. Manager: Colette Foster
Enquiries and referrals should be made to the therapy service. We operate a referral form system, available at the trust website, which is reviewed by one of the medical team at a multi-disciplinary triage meeting. The medical team are led by Dr Mike Beadsworth, consultant physician based at the Tropical and Infectious Disease Unit, Royal Liverpool Hospital. We take referrals from the north-west region.

Manchester
The Chronic Fatigue Programme, Silk House, Holyoak Street, Newton Heath, Manchester M40 1HA

Tel: 0161 219 9420 Fax: 0161 219 9477 Opening hours: Monday to Thursday 9am–4pm with answerphone available when the office is closed. Clinical lead: Gill Walsh. Team comprises a nurse and a physiotherapist. "The Chronic Fatigue Programme is a community service for adults living in Manchester who have a chronic/long term health conditions where chronic fatigue and/or chronic pain are the primary problems." "The service offers a pain course and a mindfulness course for chronic conditions, aiming to empower people to increase their self-management of pain and fatigue, reduce the day to day impact of their long-term condition on their daily life and work towards improving independence and increasing physical activity."

Norfolk and Suffolk
GP referrals to ME/CFS Service, Herbert Matthes Block, Northgate Hospital, Northgate Street, Great Yarmouth, Norfolk NR30 1BU. Tel: 01493 809 977 Fax: 01493 809970. Senior Occupational Therapist: Jo Wiggins.
Clinics at: Kirkley Mill Healthcare Centre, Lowestoft; Nelson Medical Centre, Great Yarmouth; Bowthorpe Medical Practice, Norwich; Patrick Stead Hospital, Halesworth; Stow Lodge, Stowmarket; St James Medical Practice, Kings Lynn.
"We offer an outpatient service throughout Norfolk and Suffolk, providing assessment, diagnosis, management, advice, education and support for people who have a diagnosis of CFS/ME."
"The team comprises of GP's with specialist interest (GPwSI) and knowledge of CFS/ME and Specialist Occupational Therapists (OT) and physiotherapists (PT) who are supported by administrative staff. This is via face to face appointments, email and telephone. In a small number of cases, home visits."

North Yorkshire (excluding Harrogate)
Yorkshire Fatigue Clinic, York Eco Business Centre, Amy Johnson Way, Clifton Moor, York YO30 4AG
Telephone 01904 479922 E:mail: sue@yorkshirefatigueclinic. co.uk Clinical Lead: Dr Sue Pemberton, Occupational Therapist. Other team members: Joe Bradley and Kelly Morgan, Occupational Therapists.

"We are the contracted provider for NHS assessment and rehabilitation for patients with CFS/ME in North Yorkshire, excluding adults in the Harrogate and rural area." Further information for patients, here.

Nottinghamshire
Nottingham CFS/ME Service, Mobility Centre, Hucknall Road, Nottingham. Tele: 0115 993 6628 (8.30am – 4.30pm Mon – Fri). "The Nottinghamshire adult chronic fatigue syndrome/myalgic encephalomyelitis (CFS/ME) team is based in the Mobility Centre at the City Hospital."
"It aims to help patients with mild to moderate CFS/ME to develop appropriate ways of managing their symptoms and improve their quality of life."
"Patients are offered either individual sessions or a place on an eight-week community-based group programme. Groups for up to 10 patients and their key workers run on Tuesday or Thursday mornings."

Nuneaton, Warwickshire
George Eliot Hospital, College Road, Nuneaton, Warwickshire, CV10 7DJ.
Tel: 024 7686 5212
ME/CFS service clinic days, Friday afternoons. Waiting time for initial appointment, 13 weeks. Lead clinician, Dr Vinod Patel, with multi-disciplinary team comprising occupational therapist, physiotherapist, nurse and psychologist. Dr Patel is a consultant physician in diabetes and endocrinology and Reader in Clinical Skills at Warwick Medical School..

Oxfordshire
Oxfordshire CFS/ME Service, Windrush House, Windrush Industrial Estate, Witney, Oxfordshire OX29 7DX. Tel: :01865 903 757 Fax: 01865 337 540 Email: cfs@oxfordhealth.nhs.uk Office hours: Mon-Wed 9am-1.45pm, Thurs 9am-1.30pm.
Team members: Dawn Roberts, interim manager based at the Orchard Health Centre in Banbury; Hilly Quigley and Rachael Rogers, Specialist Occupational Therapists; Glenwys Wormald, Specialist

Physiotherapist; Dr. Jean Bailey, GP with special interest in CFS/ME. Referrals should be made through GPs.

Oxford University Hospitals Fatigue Service, Churchill Hospital, Old Road, Headington, Oxford OX3 7LE. Tel: 01865 225218 Members of the team: Dr Daniel Zahl, clinical psychologist; Dr Charlie Winward, clinical specialist physiotherapist. The therapists offer NICE (National Institute for Health and Clinical Excellence) recommended treatment for ME/CFS. These are Graded Exercise Therapy (GET) and Cognitive Behavioural Therapy (CBT). These treatments focus on helping you to develop the tools to overcome your difficulties.

Peterborough and Cambridgeshire

Botolph Bridge Community Health Centre, Sugar Way, Woodston, Peterborough PE2 9QB Tel: 01733 774 583 Fax: 01733 774 514. Email: cpm-tr.CFSME@nhs.net

The Cambridgeshire and Peterborough ME/CFS Team, based in Peterborough, comprises a Specialist Nurse Practitioner and three Specialist Occupational Therapists. We offer diagnosis of ME/CFS and support in management for adults aged 17+ affected by, or suspected of having ME/CFS.

We must have a referral by a GP due to a requirement for exclusionary test results. While the team is based in Peterborough, the therapists do offer follow-up appointments at two other locations in the county.

Salford

ME/CFS Service, Salford Royal NHS Foundation Trust, Stott Lane, Salford M6 8HD. Tel: 0161 206 5153. Clinical lead: Dr Annice Mukherjee, consultant endocrinologist.

Sheffield (South Yorkshire and North Derbyshire)

Michael Carlisle Centre, Lyndhurst Road, Sheffield S11 9BJ Service manager and lead occupational therapist: Anne Nichol. Tel: 0114 226 3232 Fax: 0114 354 0124 Email: sheffieldcfsmeservice@nhs.net "This is a specialist therapy service for people affected by ME/CFS across South Yorkshire and North Derbyshire. The catchment area covers Sheffield, Rotherham, Doncaster, Barnsley, North Derbyshire County and Hardwick Clinical Commissioning Groups. The service includes

two teams – one for adults and one for children and young people."
"The service is available to individuals who have a provisional
diagnosis of CFS/ME, are registered with a GP within the region,
and who have been unable to self-manage their condition with
the advice and management provided from primary care. ME/
CFS can be a long-term and relapsing condition. Emphasis
is placed on early diagnosis and intervention to prevent the
development of more severe, complex and long-standing problems."
"Referral guidance and summary information can be found by
searching for CFS and/or ME at www.sheffieldccgportal.co.uk

Shropshire
Community Neuro Rehabilitation Team, Shropshire Rehabilitation
Centre, Lancaster Road, Harlescott, Shrewsbury SY1 3NJ.
Email for General Inquiries: cnrt@shropcom.nhs.uk
We have Occupational Therapists, Physiotherapists, Psychologists,
Speech and Language Therapists, Rehab Assistants and a Dietitian.
The named contact for the team is Dr Emma Lawrence (consultant
clinical neuropsychologist and acting manager of the Community
Neuro Rehabilitation Team), tel: 01743 453 600.

Somerset
Based at Priory House, Priory Health Park, Glastonbury Road, Wells
BA5 1XL. Contact Karen Butt, tel: 01749 836703, fax: 01749 836543.
Email: CFSME@somerset.nhs.uk
This service is provided by a small team based in Wells and uses
strategies endorsed in the NICE Clinical Guideline for ME/CFS. The
service offers assessment and treatment based on activity management
which includes pacing setting baselines and relaxation. Following
assessment, we offer up to four individual appointments with a
practitioner held in Wells or a group programme of six sessions which
are held in a number of venues across the county including Bridgwater,
Taunton and Yeovil. Telephone appointments and e-mail contact are
also available. A number of additional sessions covering particular
topics such as memory and concentration, are also provided and a
conference is held each year. The Service is open to adults aged 18
and over and a transition clinic is available for young adults currently

treated by the Paediatric Service and needing to transfer to the Adult Service. Referrals are made by a general practitioner (GP) and once accepted by our specialist doctor, appointments are usually offered within 10 weeks. The Service operates on Tuesdays, Wednesdays and Fridays each week.

South West London and Surrey (Sutton)
Tel: 0208 296 4152 (Clinical lead: Dr Amolak Bansal)
South Derbyshire
Tel: 01332 786657
Staffordshire
Tel: 01543 576609 (Correspondence to M. Wong)
The ME/CFS service is provided within the Department of Psychology (Physical Health Psychology and Rehabilitation), Cannock Chase Hospital, Brunswick Road, Cannock WS11 5XY
Stockport, Tameside and Glossop

Stockport CFS/ME Service, Floor 9 Regent House, Heaton Lane, Stockport SK4 1BS. Tel: 0161 835 6684
"The Stockport CFS/ME Service is an NHS service, offering CFS/ ME management and treatment to people registered with GPs in the Stockport and Tameside & Glossop localities."
"Referral is via a Stockport or Tameside and Glossop GP or NHS Consultant, no self-referrals; however, phone enquiries directly to our service are encouraged."
"We are a small multidisciplinary team offering home visit or clinical appointments dependent on the clients' needs and severity of illness. Our team includes an administrator, CFS/ME specialist nurses, physiotherapists, occupational therapist and a cognitive behavioural therapist (CBT)."
"Our management approach includes pacing and activity management, relaxation techniques, managing stress, graded activity, guidance on sleep problems, managing setbacks, coping strategies and goal setting, and CBT. We work collaboratively with our clients to better manage the variety of symptoms associated with CFS/ME, and improve quality of life."

Sussex-wide

Haywards Heath Health Centre, Heath Road, Haywards Heath, West Sussex RH16 3BB. To contact the administrator, Jenny Goldsmith, please phone 01444 475 799. Email: jenny.goldsmith@nhs.net "The clinical lead doctor also runs clinics in Brighton. The service also offers group and individual treatments at out-patient clinics in Eastbourne. Referrals are accepted from GPs following completion of the service referral form including comprehensive blood-screening tests." "The majority of patients take part in the multi-disciplinary out-patient group self-management programme. The course covers topics such as rest and activity management, sleep management, graded exercise (activity) and lifestyle management within a cognitive behavioural framework. The group is reviewed after three months."

Swindon and Wiltshire CFS/ME Service

Eldene Health Centre, Eldene, Swindon SN3 3RZ. "This service has a GP with a special interest as the clinical lead. Others in the team – all with a special interest in ME/CFS – are a physiotherapist, an occupational therapist, a psychologist and a dietitian." "The service sees people 1:1 or in group sessions and offers a variety of techniques to help people with the illness manage their difficulties and improve their quality of life. Courses are held periodically through the year. Referral to the service is through GPs only."

Tees Valley

The ME/CFS Team, Department of Infectious Diseases and Travel Medicine, James Cook University Hospital, South Tees Foundation NHS Trust, Marton Road, Middlesborough TS4 3BW, tel: 01642 835898. "The team includes: Dr John Williams clinical lead/consultant physician, Dr Brendan McCarron consultant physician, Dr David R Chadwick consultant physician, Sister Amanda McGough specialist nurse, Dr Alison Woods senior clinical psychologist, Mrs Angela Park specialist physiotherapist. Referrals to the clinical psychologist and specialist physiotherapist can only be made by the CFS/ME team. There is no direct access to these services at present."

Newcastle, North Tynside and Northumberland

Molineux Street NHS Centre, Newcastle upon Tyne, NE6 1SG. Tel: 0191 213 8823. Email: jeanette.welch@nuth.nhs.uk
Office hours 8.15am – 4.15pm, Wednesday and Thursday; 9.00am – 12.45pm Friday.
"The team working with CFS/ME patients in our area has a range of experience, and includes: consultants in immunology, and infectious and tropical medicine, clinical psychologists who carry out the initial psychological assessment, and work with patients whose condition has impacted on their physical and psychological well-being, cognitive behavioural therapists, and physiotherapists."

South of Tyne Chronic Fatigue Syndrome Service

Chester Lodge Sunderland Royal Hospital Kayll Road Sunderland Tel: 0191 541 0045. The Head of the Psychology Service is Dr Tony Wells.
"Referrals to the South of Tyne Chronic Fatigue Syndrome Service are accepted from GPs located across the Gateshead, South Tyneside and Sunderland geographical areas."
"The aim of this service is to provide assessment, enhanced condition management and symptomatic treatment, for people who have chronic fatigue syndrome (CFS). We hope to assist in the prevention of longer term and more severe symptoms by providing early intervention."

Wiltshire South

Tel: 01225 465941 (ext 202)
Castle Street Surgery, Salisbury SP1 3SP
Clinical leads: Katy McCarthy, specialist occupational therapist, and Dr Graham Jaggard, GP with a special interest.

Worcestershire

Chronic Fatigue Syndrome Service, Malvern Community Hospital, 185 Worcester Road, Malvern, Worcestershire WR14 1EX. Tel: 01684 612 671 This is a part-time service with admin hours as follows: Tues-Wed 8am-1pm, Thurs 8am-12noon. Email: WHCNHS.chronicfatigue@nhs.net
"We are a specialist part-time service that delivers support and treatment to people with CFS/ME within community settings across Worcestershire."
"The main aspect of our treatment is our Managing Lifestyles

Group programme. This offers patients the opportunity to learn more about the ways in which they can manage their condition, with the aim of improving functional independence and quality of life." "The group teaches skills in sleep management, pacing, relaxation and mindfulness, and communication, as well as many further topics. We find that the majority of our patients benefit greatly from this programme and particularly find that meeting and building relationships with other group members helps to reduce the isolation that is so commonly felt as a result of the condition."

Part 3
Children and Adolescent NHS ME/CFS Specialist Services in England

Bath Paediatric ME/CFS Service
Children's Centre, Royal United Hospital, Combe Park, Bath BA1 3NG. Tel: 01225 821 340
Team administrator; Heather Hill
The Bath paediatric ME/CFS service provides local, regional and national assessment and treatment for over 150 children and young people each year. It is now open to the 'choose and book' appointment system run by the NHS. This means that children or adolescents anywhere in the country should have access to their outpatient service for advice on either diagnosis or management through a GP referral.

Brighton and Hove
Paediatric CFS/ME Service for Brighton and Hove, Seaside View Child Development Centre, Brighton General Hospital, Elm Grove, Brighton BN2 3EW, tel: 01273 265 780 Email: SC-Tr.BGH-seasideview@nhs.net Team members: Dr Victoria Thornton (clinical psychologist), Julia Krikman (occupational therapist), Claire Neyland (team administrator). The team meets together only once a week on Wednesdays so it may take a few days to return phone calls.

Cambridgeshire and Peterborough

The Children's Community Nursing Teams Nightingale Court, Ida Darwin Fulbourn Cambridge CB1 5EE Tel: 01223 884335 Fax: 01223 884299 The lead paediatrician is Dr David Vickers. This a small community team based at the Ida Darwin unit, Fulbourn, who provide a specialist service to children and young people up to the age of 19 years with CSF/ ME, who are registered with a GP and attend school in Cambridgeshire and Peterborough.

Cornwall and the Isles of Scilly

Cornwall and Isles of Scilly CFS/ME Service, The Lighthouse, Royal Cornwall Hospitals Trust. Truro. TR1 3LJ 01872 252935. New services for children and young people under 16 have been commissioned by Kernow Clincial Commissioning Group for patients registered with a GP in the county.

Cumbria (North)

Children's Community Team, Cockermouth Cottage Hospital, Isel Road, Cockermouth, Cumbria CA13 9HT
Tel: 01900 324 131 Mob: 07789 925 705
Service lead: Laura Wilson, children and young people's CFS/ME practitioner.

Devon

Tel: 01392 208614
Royal Devon and Exeter Hospital
Paediatrician: Dr James Hart, Occupational therapist: Helga Gore.

Dorset

CFS/ME Service for Children and Young People, Children's Centre, Damers Road, Dorchester, DT1 2LB.
Tel: 01305 253148 Email: dorset.cfs@dchft.nhs.uk
Assessment and treatment is available to all children living in Dorset with appointments offered locally. Limited domiciliary visits are available if required for those unable to attend an out-patient appointment.

East and North Hertfordshire
East and North Hertfordshire NHS Trust Chronic Fatigue Syndrome Service for Children and Young People, Children and Adolescent Unit, Lister Hospital, Coreys Mill Lane, Stevenage, Hertfordshire, SG1 4AB. Tele:01438284235.Fax:01438284812.Email:cfspaeds.enh-tr@nhs.net We are a Specialist Team comprising: Dr Deborah Gale, Specialist Clinical Psychologist; Janey Readman, Specialist Nurse; Lisa Ackerman, Specialist Physiotherapist.

Liverpool
CFS/ME Service Alder Hey Children's Hospital, Eaton Road, Liverpool, L12 2AP
Tel: 0151 228 4811 (ext 3803)
"This is a general paediatrician led multidisciplinary team (MDT) including senior physiotherapist, CFS/ME specialist nurse, psychologist, consultant psychiatrist and a medical secretary. We provide both diagnostic and therapeutic services to children and young people with this condition coming from Liverpool, Knowsly and Sefton areas."

Manchester
Harrington Building, Royal Manchester Children's Hospital, Oxford Road, Manchester M13 9WL.
Tele: 0161 701 4516 Email: cfs.me@cmft.nhs.uk
Coordinating clinician: Alexandra Woore.

London

Great Ormond Street Hospital
Tel: 0207 813 8541

University College Hospital
235 Euston Road London NW1 2BUU
Tel: 08451 555000
Consultants: Jo Begent and Terry Segal
The UCLH adolescent ME/CFS service provides local and tertiary assessment and treatment, as in and out patients between the

ages of 13 to 19 years old. The service is delivered by a multidisciplinary team which includes nurse specialist, OT, physiotherapist, psychologist and doctors.

Nottinghamshire
Children's Service, C Floor, South Block, Office 3086, Queens Medical Centre, Nottingham NG7 2HU
Tel: 0115 924 9924 (ext 66282)
Clinical co-ordinator and Specialist Occupational Therapist at the Nottingham Children's Hospital: Jacqui McIntyre, email: Jacqui.McIntyre@nuh.nhs.uk
Working days – Monday to Thursday. Referrals must be made by a consultant paediatrician.

South Yorkshire and North Derbyshire
See Sheffield entry in 'Adult Services'.

North of Tyne
Dr Caroline Grayson, Community paediatrician, Newcastle Hospitals NHS Trust, Royal Victoria Infirmary, Queen Victoria Road, Newcastle upon Tyne NE1 4LP, Telephone: 0191 282 5517, Email: gavin.spickett@nuth.nhs.uk

South of Tyne and Wear
Department of Paediatrics, City Hospitals Sunderland NHS Foundation Trust, Kayll Road, Sunderland SR4 7TP, Tel: 0191 5656256 ext: 42899 Fax: 0191 5699219 Email: neil.hopper@chsft.nhs.uk
Clinical lead: Dr Neil Hopper, consultant paediatrician. We see which sees children and young people up to the age of 18 with CFS. We cover Sunderland, South Tyneside and Gateshead and comprise two paediatricians, one paediatric physio and one psychologist.

Part 4
NHS ME/CFS Specialist services in Scotland

Astley Ainslie Hospital

Department of Clinical Psychology, Astley Ainslie Hospital, 133 Grange Loan, Edinburgh EH9 2HL. Open only on Thursdays and Fridays. Tel: 0131 537 9139.

This is a Lothian-wide service for patients with a diagnosis of ME/CFS, who are well enough to attend the service. The service was set up as a two-year pilot starting in November 2012 but has since been granted a year's extension to run until the end of November 2015. It is based in the hospital's pain management service and is run by specialist physiotherapy and applied psychology staff.

Glasgow

NHS Centre for Integrative Care, 1053 Great Western Road, Glasgow G12 0XQ, Tel: 0141 211 1600. Clinical lead: Dr David Reilly.

Fife

Scotland's only specialist nurse-led service for patients with ME/CFS is at the LadyBank Clinic, Commercial Road, Ladybank, Fife KY15 7JS, tel: 01337 832 123, email: keithanderson1@nhs.netIt is run by Keith Anderson, a qualified psychotherapist and CBT therapist. Mr Anderson recently gave a talk to Edinburgh ME Self Help Group;

Stornaway, Western Isles

A Fatigue Management Programme was opened in May 2011 at the Western Isles Hospital in Stornoway to help people with fatigue to explore the reasons for the fatigue and equip them with the techniques to manage the problem better. A video link to Uist and Barra Hospital may be set up, if there is a demand for it. The Western Isles, with a population of about 26,000 people, has no specialist ME/CFS service. To inquire about joining the programme, please contact Elaine Smith, Occupational Therapy Department, tel: 01851 708287, or email elaine.smith1@nhs.net who will send you an application form.

NHS SPECIALIST SERVICES IN WALES We are building up a picture of specialist NHS services for adults and children with M.E. in Wales. If you know of any good services, please let us know. If you have any tried any services, your feedback will be most welcome.

North Wales ME/CFS Service
The Quay Clinic, Fron Road, Connah's Quay, Deeside CH5 4PJ. Callers to the building should press the option for 'Bloods/Reception' and ask for the ME/CFS Clinic. Tel: 01244 813 486 Fax: 01244 830883 (This service takes referrals from the east of North Wales. Staff: Simon Neal, clinical psychologist; Penny Cowley, head of dietetics; Chris Watson, superintendent physiotherapist).

CFS/ME Service (North Wales)
CFS/ME Service, Betsi Cadwaladr University Health Board, Cartref, Cartref, Ysbyty Bryn y Neuadd, Conwy, LL33 0HH
Tel: 01248 682 843 (Clinic answerphone 01248 682 874)
Clinical lead: Dr Helen Lyon Jones, consultant clinical psychologist.
Dr Meirion Llewellyn at the Royal Gwent Hospital in Newport sees some ME/CFS patients. Tel: 01633 234234
Pain and Fatigue Management Centre
Bronllys Hospital, Brecon, Powys LD3 0LU.
For referrals or more information, contact Margaret Davies, the office manager, tel: 01874 712 499.

Part 5:

NHS ME/CFS Specialist Services in Northern Ireland
The care pathways for people with ME/CFS in Northern Ireland are not well established and there is no specialist service for people with ME/CFS in the Province.
Thanks to Mrs Antoinette Christie, from ME Support in Northern Ireland, who has made available part of the text of a letter she has received in response to inquiries made to both the Minister of Health and the Assembly's Health Committee:

"There has never been a Commissioned service for CFS/ME in the Belfast Health and social care trust. Dr Welby Henry, a consultant physician provided a CFS/ME clinic in Belfast City Hospital since at least 1986 on a special interest basis. Dr Henry has now retired.

The Belfast Trust and the health and social care board are currently discussing how best to accommodate the gap in services following Dr Henry's retirement."

Mrs Joan McParland, of Hope4MEandFibro Northern Ireland, wrote on 20 November 2016:

"A Condition Management Programme for ME/CFS has been operating in the Northern Trust for a number of years. We met with the staff a few months ago and they confirmed they are offering self-management advice only, not GET as was previously thought. GPs can refer patients in Northern Trust catchment area."

Printed in Great Britain
by Amazon